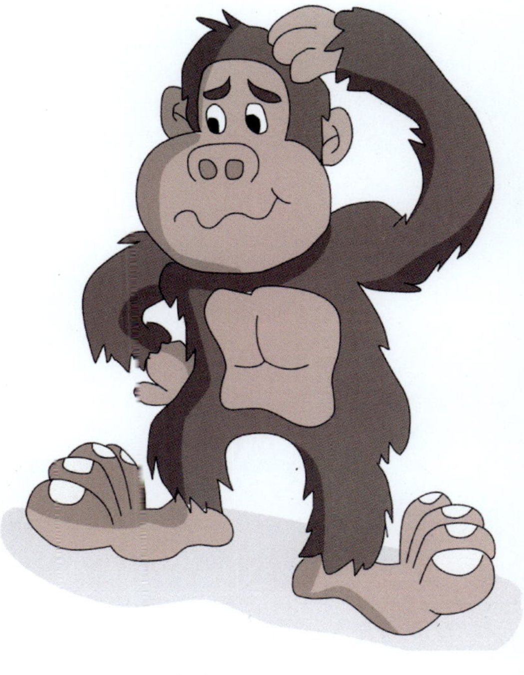

## Acknowledgements

**Kimberley Cheung** Contributor
**Andrew Chan** App Developer
**Stanley Cheng** Mentor
**Aissa Bautista** Artist
**LaunchBox Program** at Trinity College Dublin

Special thanks to our families and friends for supporting us through this endeavour.

## Disclaimer

This book is designed for educational use only and should not be used in the medical diagnosis, treatment, or management of patients. This book contains satire and parody and no infringement of copyright is intended.

**www.visuallearner.net**

**ISBN-13: 978-1502363800**
**ISBN-10: 1502363801**

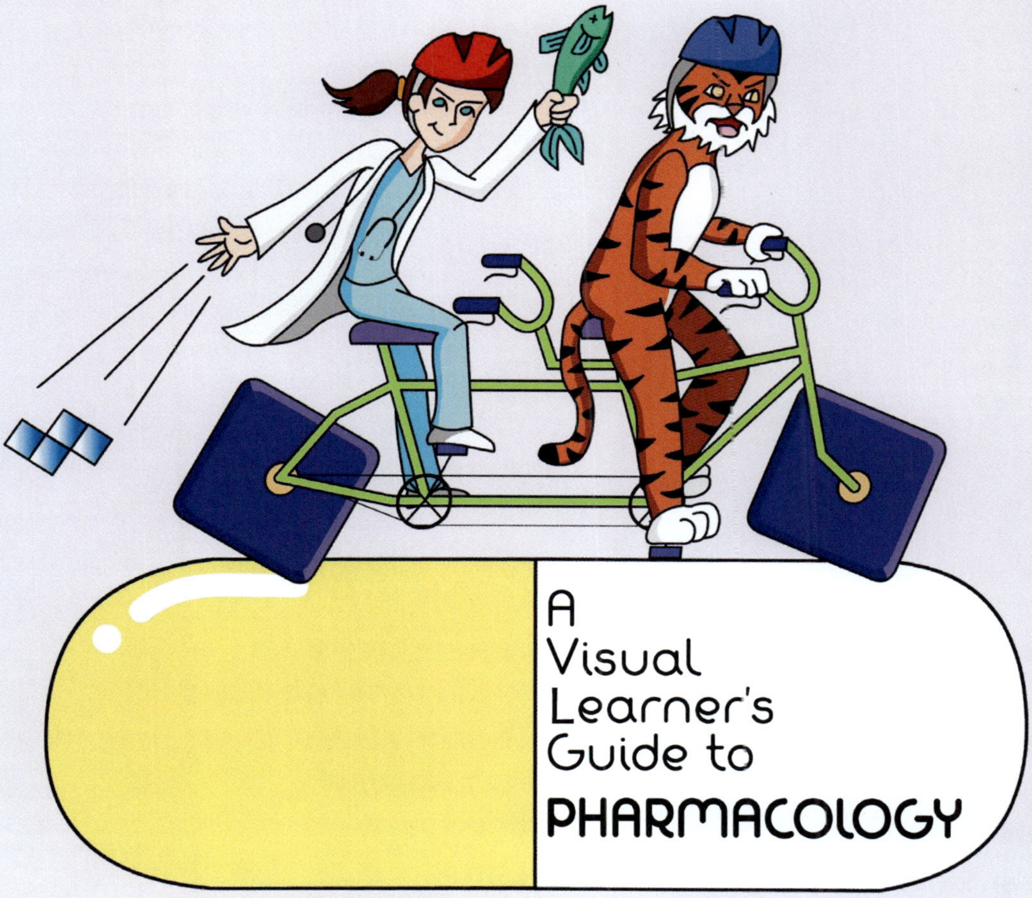

# A Visual Learner's Guide to PHARMACOLOGY

**FIRST EDITION**


**CREATED BY**
**DR. PETER WU**
**DR. EDWIN CHU**
**& PATRICK WU**

# TABLE OF CONTENTS

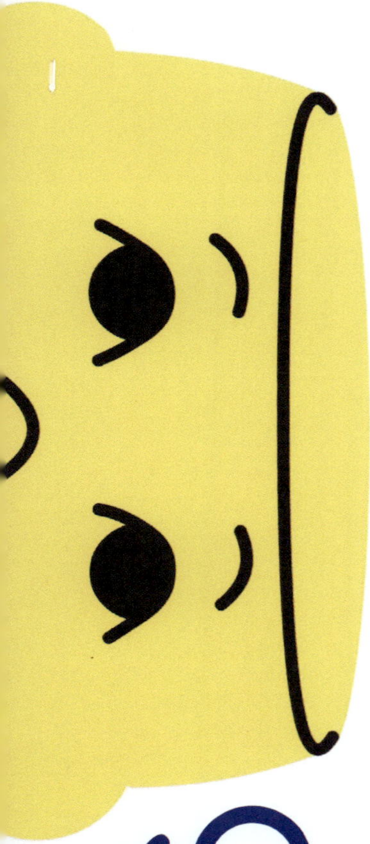

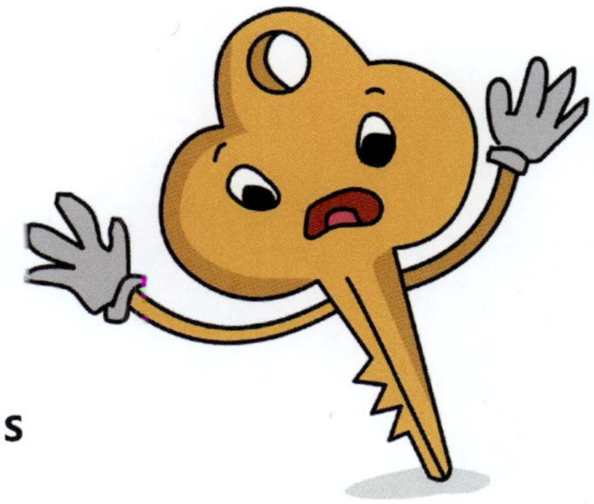

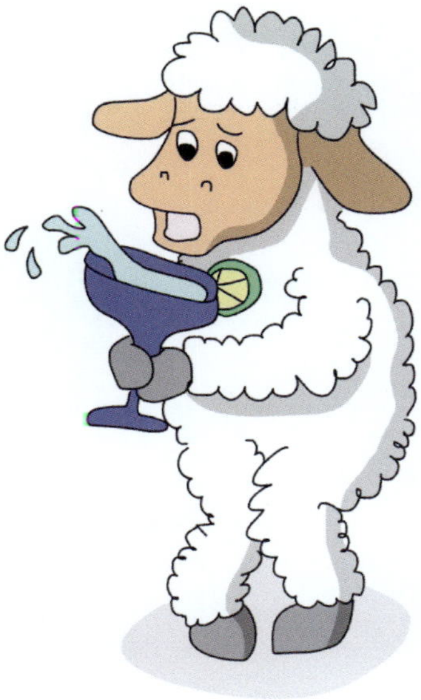

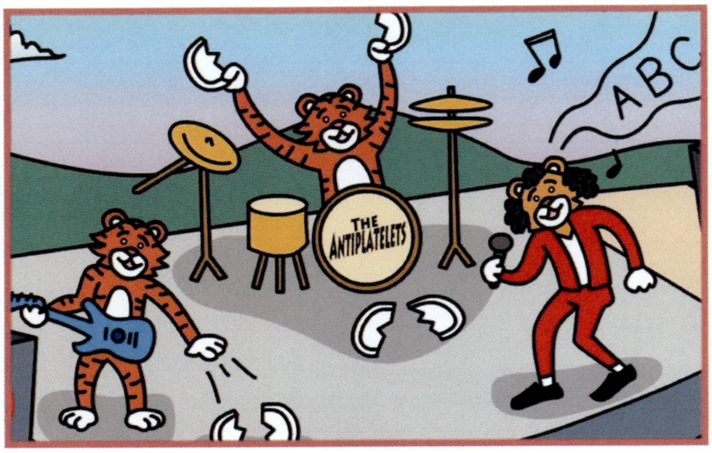


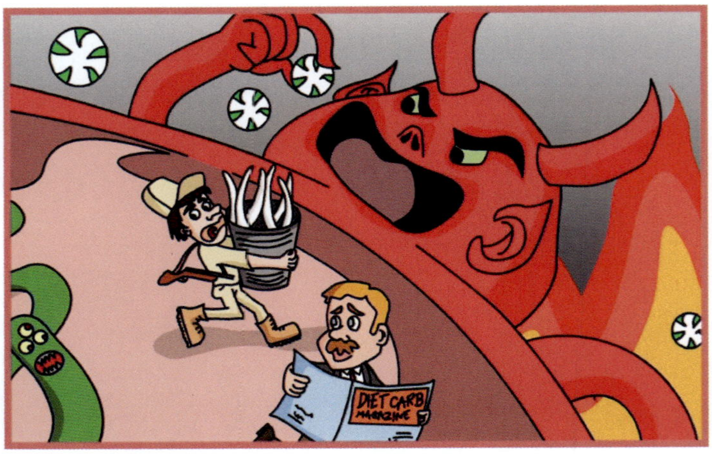


# INTRODUCTION: THE VISUAL AGE

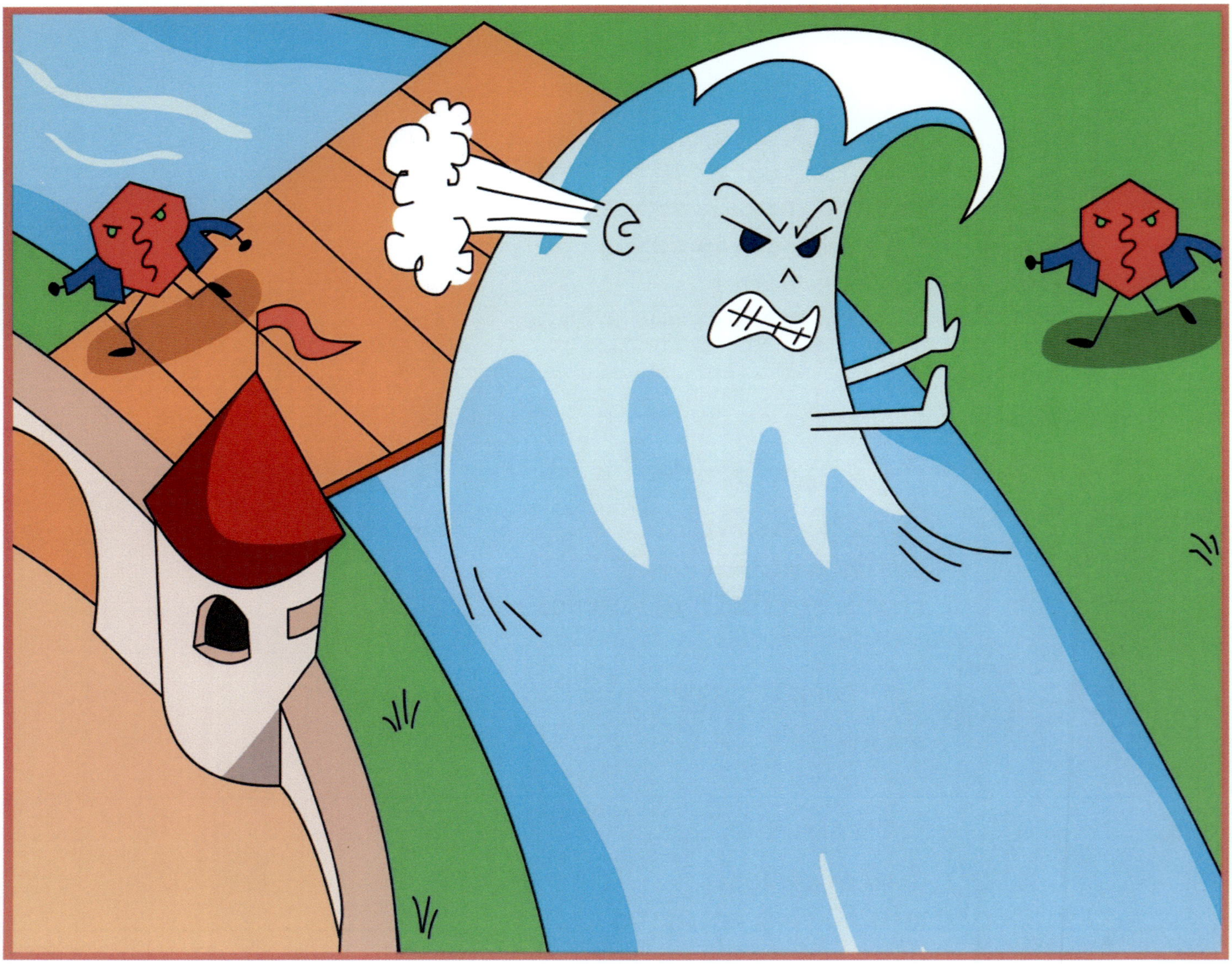

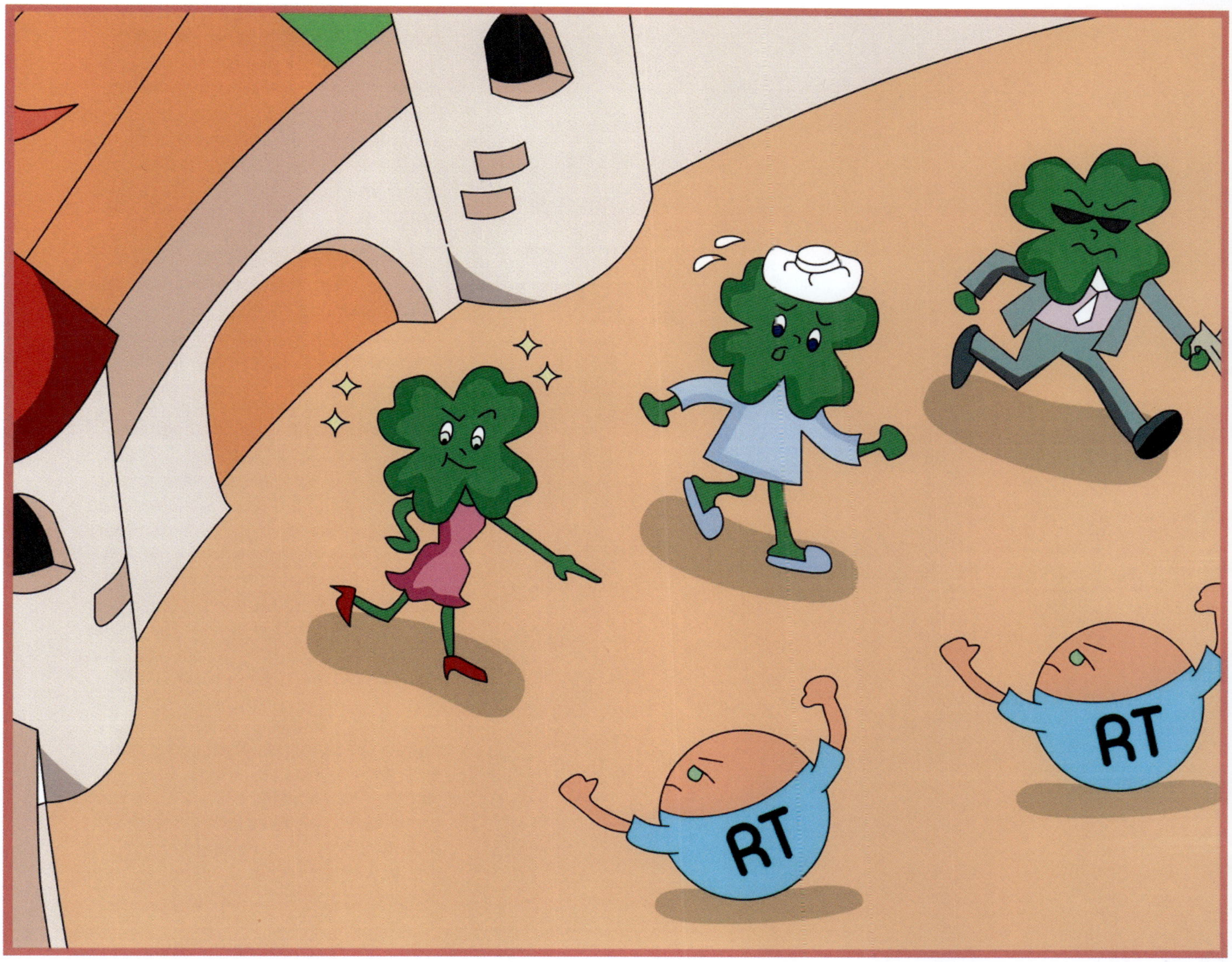


**WELCOME TO THE FIRST EDITION OF THE VISUAL LEARNER'S GUIDE TO PHARMACOLOGY.** This book was created with the student in mind, and its purpose is to make studying more efficient and effective. We would like to thank all our artists and writers for the countless hours spent creating this project, and our families for the patience and financial support in this endeavour.

Pharmacology is a huge branch of medicine, with hundreds of difficult drug names and concepts. Students are given the tough task of memorizing large amounts of information in a short amount of time, and often look for supplemental study aids for help. An important part of these aids are mnemonics, which are devices that aid memorization. Typically, text-based mnemonics have been used as they are the easy to create and implement.

Let's take an example found in psychiatry with a well known mnemonic for the symptoms of depression: "SIG-E-CAPS". "S" for changes in sleep pattern, "I" for interest loss, "G" for feelings of guilt, "E" for energy loss, "C" for concentration, "A" for appetite changes, "P" for psychomotor disturbances,

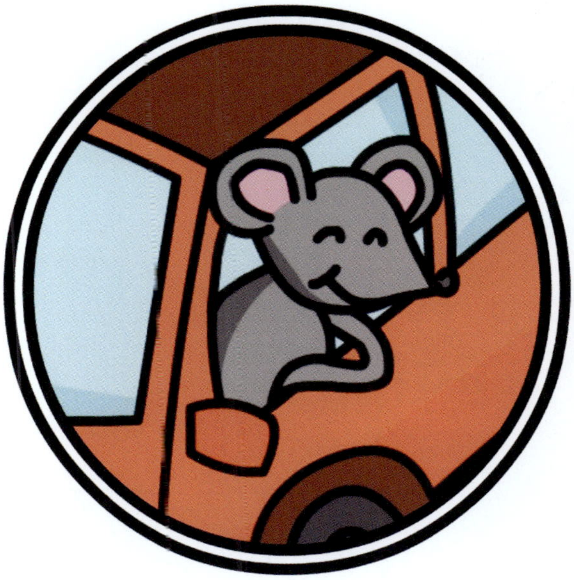

*"Van-Mice"*
**Vancomycin**

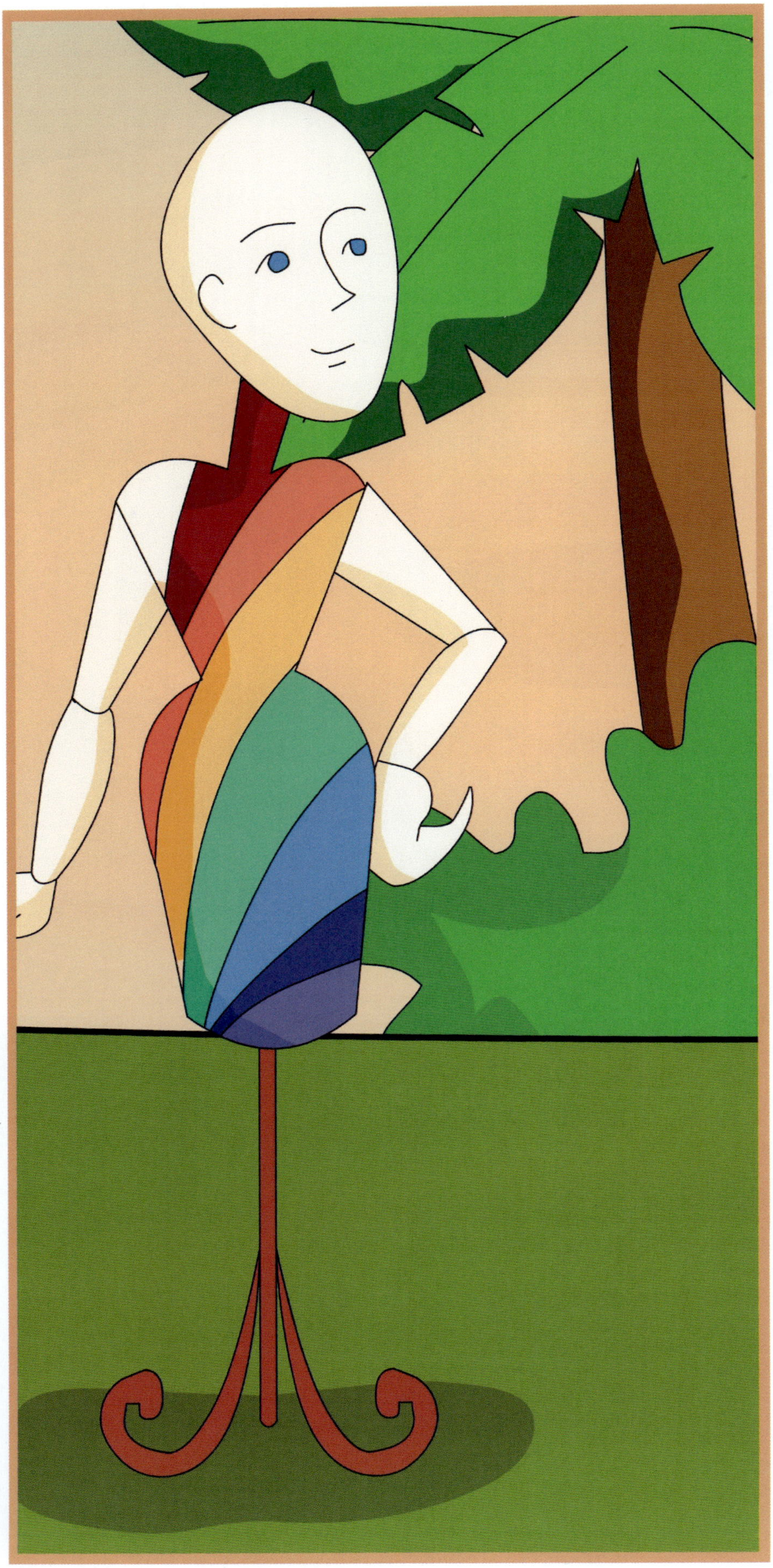

and “S” for suicidal ideation. A mnemonic like this is designed to help students remember all key points, by providing a memory trigger in the form of the first letter of each symptom. The idea would be that the student would just have to remember the words “SIG-E-CAPS”, and the letters would prompt the brain to remember each symptom.

Mnemonics are used by students because they work. However, with multiple word-mnemonics with the same letters, it becomes more and more difficult to remember what each letter means.

We’ve taken mnemonics to the next level by adding a visual component. Empirical research suggests that the majority of the population have a visual learning style, and studies have shown that absorption and retention of material are significantly improved in students who revise in a format that complements their learning style. So we’ve combined the most important learning style with the power of mnemonics, to bring you a new tool in learning: “visual mnemonics”.

Our book is designed to help you memorize all the important drug names and classes. Each character that is created represents a specific drug. Characters are grouped into pictures that represent their drug category. Remember the pictures, and you can remember all the drugs that are part of a specific category.

It’s important to realize that this book should be used as supplemental material to your course material, rather than a substitute. And that if you want to succeed, than time, effort, and concentration are needed, even with this study aid.

We hope that you find this book useful and that it helps you succeed in your studies. Please leave comments and suggestions to **visualmnemonics@gmail.com**, and visit our website at **visuallearner.net** for more information and all our videos.

*With love,*

**Visual Learner Studios**

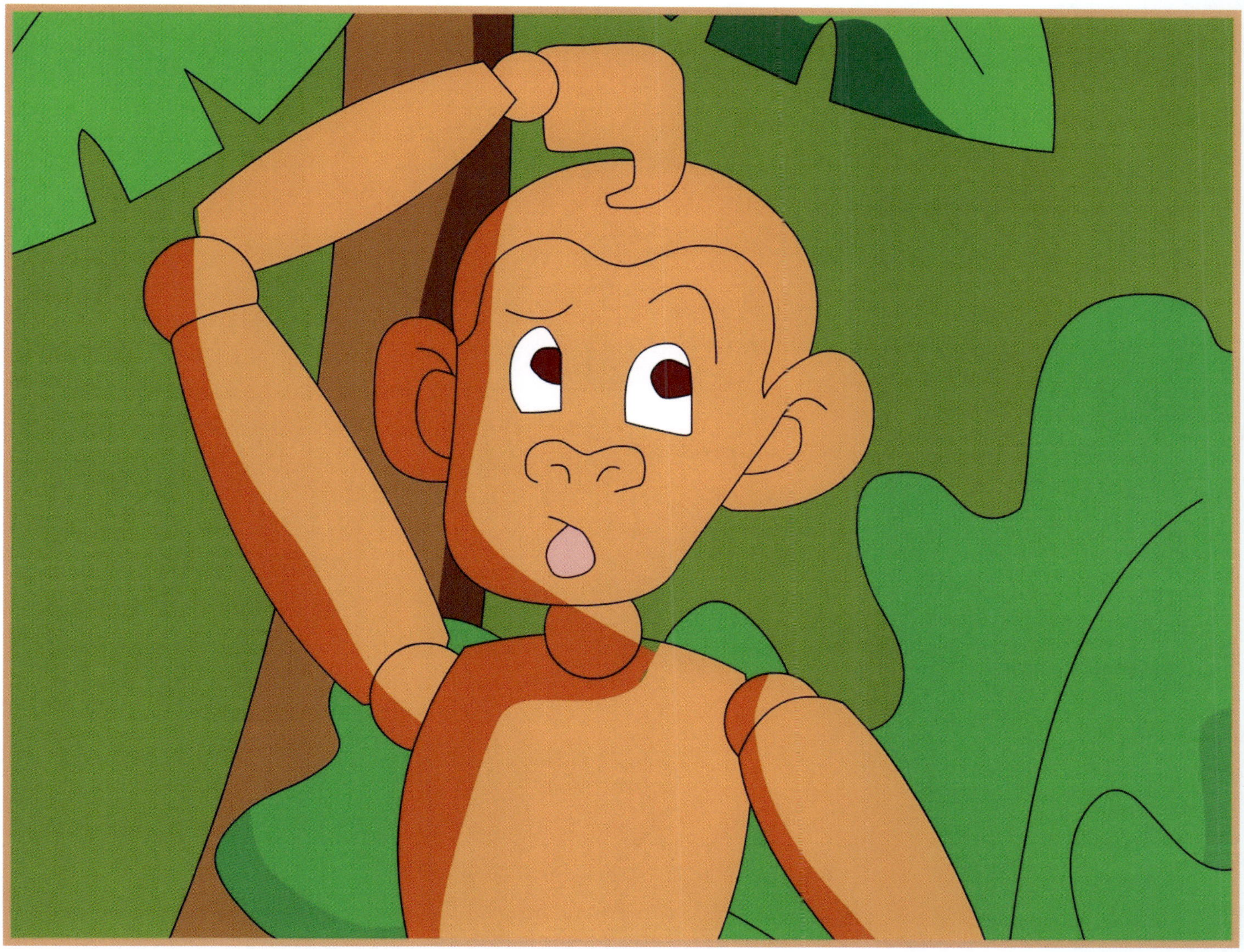

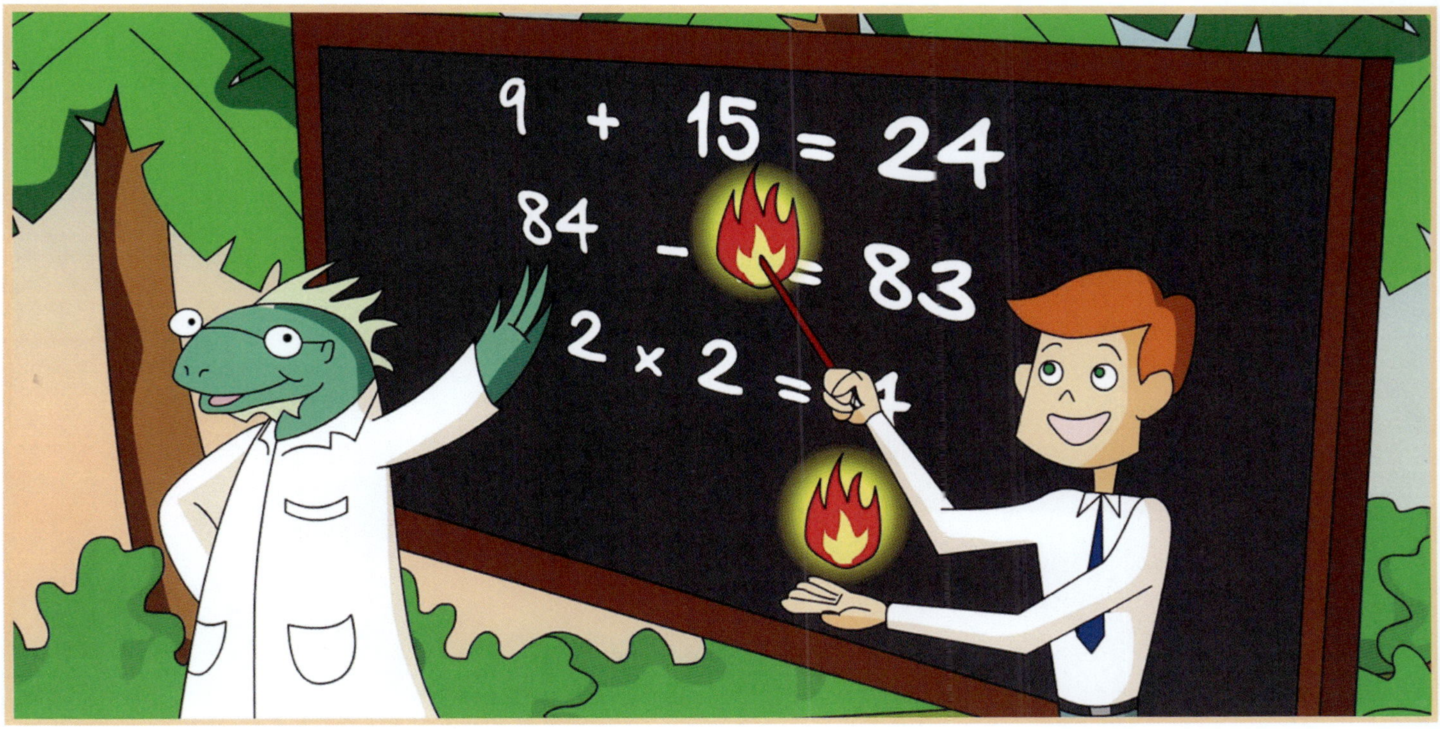
9 + 15 = 24
84 -
= 83
2 × 2 =

# ANTIHISTAMINES

## HOW TO USE THIS BOOK

Each topic includes written information and a memorable vignette with unique characters depicting important medications.

Remembering drug names is easy when you use the power of visual learning!

drug sensitivity rashes, pruritis, insomnia,

### INDICATIONS

Look for symbol:

ms of
hroat.
ory and
aries

In ... lls in connective tissu ... of the stomach and plays a role i ... on of gastric acid.

Antihistamines a ... ated into first- and second-generation classes. First-generation antihista ... an cross the blood brain barrier to a much greater extent than second-generation ... g to increa ... erefore they are referred to as "drowsy", while second-generation a ... drowsy".

Antihistamines are used to tre ... according to its target receptors. There are ... his ... n body, but the most commonly used ant ... and histamine-2 (H2) receptors.

H1 receptors are fou ... mooth muscle cells and the tuberomammillary nucle ... nists can be sub-classified according to their selectivity ... an ... eration.

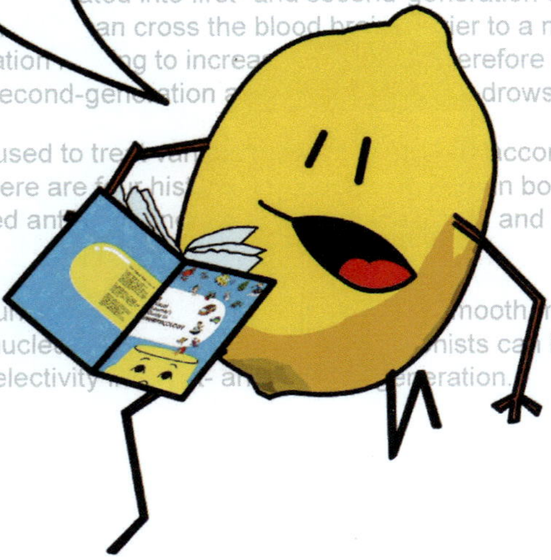

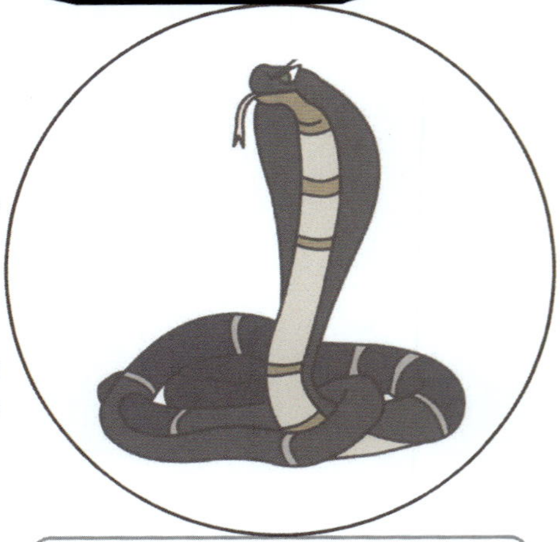

The "HSSSsss" reminds you this picture is for Anti-"HSSSsss"-tamines [antihistamines].

### KEY REMINDER

Each picture contains a key reminder of the topic, which serves as a trigger for memory.

## H1 First ...

The firs ... *chlorph* ... non-sel ... central ... sicknes ...

They ... alpha-ad ... Side effe ... itchiness, v ... bronchoconstri ...

### SPECIFIC DRUG INFORMATION

Find drug methods of action, side effects, and other frequently appearing exam material here to supplement your class teaching.

## H1 Second-Generation Antihi ... nes

Second-generation H1 antagonists, such ... ***fexofenadine***, ***loratadine***, and ***cetirizine*** specifically target peripheral H1 receptors instead of the H1 receptors in the central nervous system. This sub-group of drug is generally well-tolerated and cause very few side effects.

## ... Receptor Antagonists

*... or more information on H2 receptor antagonists and their ... ual mnemonics, see chapter on* ***Peptic Ulcer Disease.***

H2 receptors are found mostly in the stomach lining. H2 antagonists act mainly in the peripheral tissues. Specifically, they bind to H2 receptors located on the surface of parietal cells responsible for the secretion of gastric acid. As a result, they are able to decrease gastric acid secretion.

In clinical practice, H2 antagonists are used for the treatment and prevention of gastroesophageal reflux disease, gastritis and peptic ulcer disease.

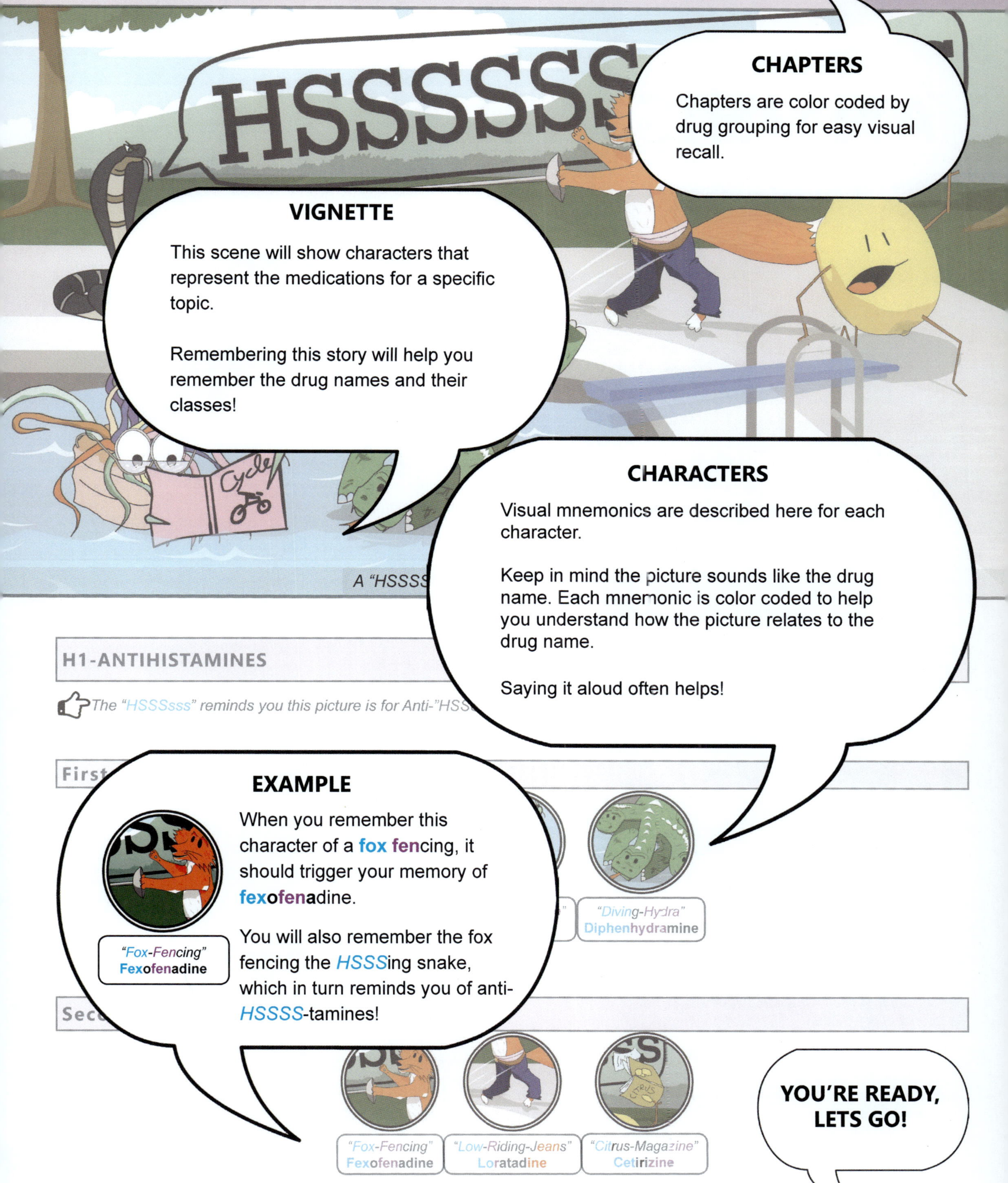

HSSSSSS
A "HSSSS
H1-ANTIHISTAMINES
The "HSSSsss" reminds you this picture is for Anti-"HSS
First
"Diving-Hydra"
Diphenhydramine
Sec
"Fox-Fencing"
Fexofenadine
"Low-Riding-Jeans"
Loratadine
"Citrus-Magazine"
Cetirizine


**CHAPTERS**

Chapters are color coded by drug grouping for easy visual recall.

**VIGNETTE**

This scene will show characters that represent the medications for a specific topic.

Remembering this story will help you remember the drug names and their classes!

**CHARACTERS**

Visual mnemonics are described here for each character.

Keep in mind the picture sounds like the drug name. Each mnemonic is color coded to help you understand how the picture relates to the drug name.

Saying it aloud often helps!

**EXAMPLE**

"Fox-Fencing"
Fexofenadine

When you remember this character of a **fox fen**cing, it should trigger your memory of **fexofen**adine.

You will also remember the fox fencing the *HSSS*ing snake, which in turn reminds you of anti-*HSSSS*-tamines!

**YOU'RE READY, LETS GO!**

# ANTIHISTAMINES

**Indications for H1-antihistamines:** hay fever, urticaria, drug sensitivity rashes, pruritis, insomnia.

**ANTIHISTAMINES** are medications used to relieve or prevent symptoms of allergies such as hives, rashes, nasal congestion, and itchy eyes, skin, or throat. They target histamine, a chemical compound involved in immuno-modulatory and pro-inflammatory responses that increase the permeability of blood capillaries allowing white blood cells to combat foreign substances in the body.

In allergic reactions, histamine is released by mast cells and basophils in connective tissues. It is also stored in the enterochromaffin-like (ECL) cells of the stomach and plays a role in the secretion of gastric acid.

Antihistamines are segregated into first- and second-generation classes. First-generation antihistamines can cross the blood brain barrier to a much greater extent than second-generation leading to increased sedation, therefore they are referred to as "drowsy", while second-generation are considered "non-drowsy".

Antihistamines are used to treat various medical conditions according to its target receptors. There are four histamine receptors in human body, but the most commonly used antihistamines target histamine-1 (H1) and histamine-2 (H2) receptors.

H1 receptors are found on endothelial cells, mast cells, smooth muscle cells, and the tuberomammillary nucleus of the brain. The H1 antagonists can be sub-classified according to their selectivity into first- and second-generation.

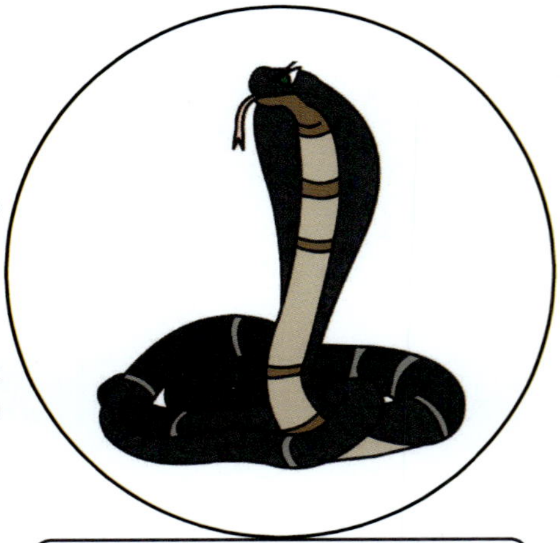

The "HSSSsss" reminds you this picture is for Anti-"HSSSsss"-tamines [antihistamines].

### H1 First-Generation Antihistamines

The first generation H1 antagonists such as ***chlorphenamine***, ***cyclizine***, and ***diphenhydramine*** are non-selective, in that they act on both peripheral and central receptors. Specifically, they block the action of histamine at the H1 receptor. They are used to treat allergies, motion sickness, and can be used as a sleeping aid. Side effects of H1 antagonists include drowsiness, skin itchiness, vasodilation, hypotension, tachycardia, and bronchoconstriction.

### H1 Second-Generation Antihistamines

Second-generation H1 antagonists, such as ***fexofenadine***, ***loratadine***, and ***cetirizine***, specifically target peripheral H1 receptors instead of the H1 receptors in the central nervous system. This sub-group of drug is generally well-tolerated and cause very few side effects.

### H2 Receptor Antagonists

*For more information on H2 receptor antagonists and their visual mnemonics, see chapter on peptic ulcer disease (page 37).*

H2 receptors are found mostly in the stomach lining. H2 antagonists act mainly in the peripheral tissues. Specifically, they bind to H2 receptors located on the surface of parietal cells responsible for the secretion of gastric acid. As a result, they are able to decrease gastric acid secretion.

In clinical practice, H2 antagonists are used for the treatment and prevention of gastroesophageal reflux disease, gastritis and peptic ulcer disease.

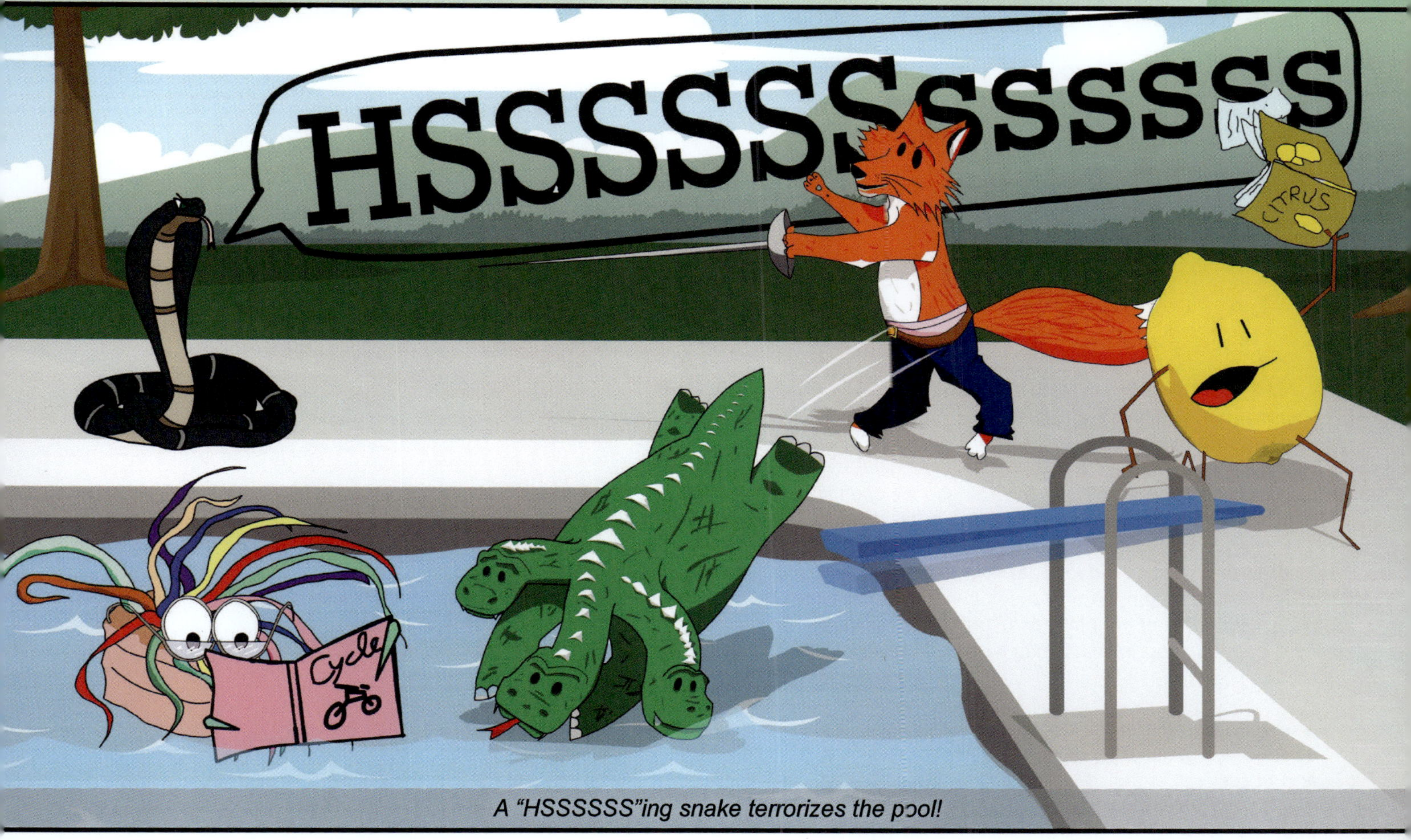


*A "HSSSSSS"ing snake terrorizes the pool!*

## H1-ANTIHISTAMINES

👉 *The "HSSSsss" reminds you this picture is for Anti-"HSSSsss"-tamines [antihistamines].*

### First Generation

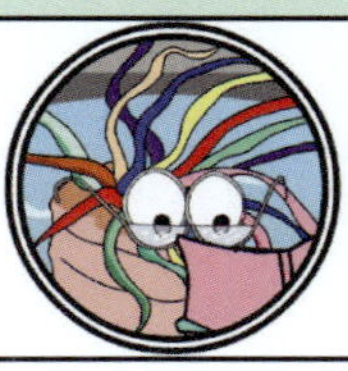

"Colorful-Anemone"
**Chlorphenamine**

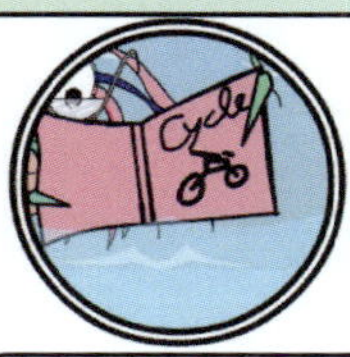

"Cycle-Magazine"
**Cyclizine**

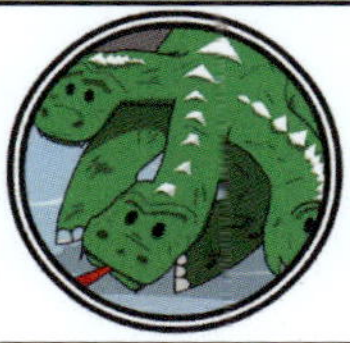

"Diving-Hydra"
**Diphenhydramine**

### Second Generation

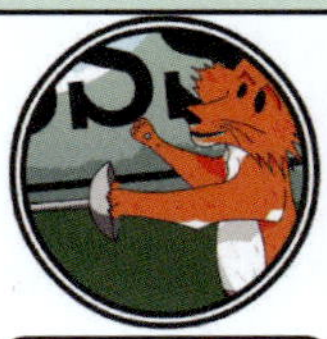

"Fox-Fencing"
**Fexofenadine**

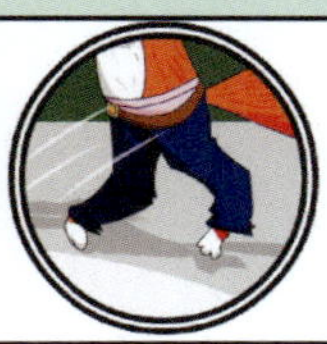

"Low-Riding-Jeans"
**Loratadine**

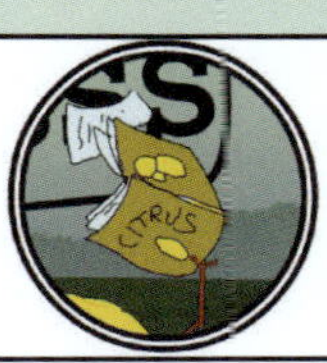

"Citrus-Magazine"
**Cetirizine**

# ANAPHYLAXIS

**Indications for anaphylaxis drugs:** anaphylaxis (shortness of breath, swelling lips/tongue/throat, etc).

**ANAPHYLAXIS** is a life-threatening allergic reaction that warrants immediate treatment. Anaphylaxis is classified as a type I hypersensitivity reaction, meaning that there is an exaggerated response to an allergen.

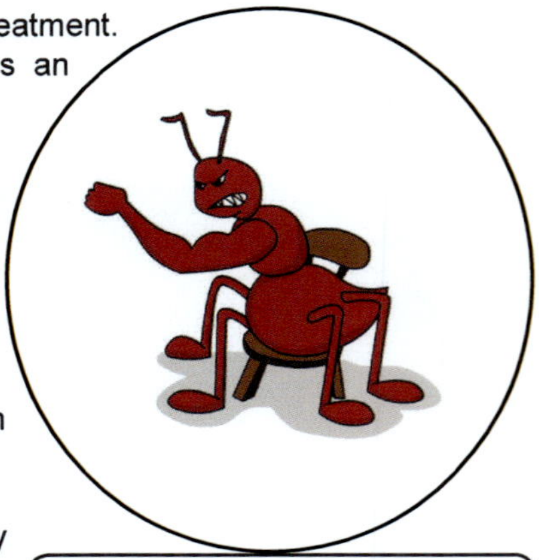

The ant-flexing reminds you this picture is about anaphylaxis!

Anaphylaxis is triggered by the release of chemical mediators from white blood cells that are involved in allergic reactions such as mast cells, basophils, and eosinophils. The allergic reaction can be triggered by either a immunological or non-immunological mechanism, and avoidance of allergen triggers remains the gold standard for the prevention of anaphylaxis. Causes can include allergies to food, medications, and insect bites. The onset of anaphylaxis usually falls between minutes to hours. It is characterized by a sudden drop in blood pressure, difficulty breathing, swelling of the throat, and skin rashes.

Since patients who suffer from anaphylaxis experience shortness of breath, oxygen therapy through a high-flow mask is used to enhance oxygen delivery to the respiring tissues and to prevent further deterioration of the condition. Intubation may also be necessary if respiratory obstruction is likely to occur. It is preferable to keep the patient in a lying position to ensure blood does not stagnate in the lower extremities.

## Epinephrine

The first line treatment for anaphylaxis is intramuscular ***epinephrine*** (adrenaline) to relieve breathing difficulties and increase blood pressure. The intramuscular route of administration is preferred over subcutaneous because it has a quicker onset of action and is the best option in an emergency situation.

***Epinephrine*** causes vasoconstriction through the binding of alpha-1 adrenergic receptors, increasing peripheral resistance and systemic arterial blood pressure. Furthermore, it decreases the permeability of blood vessels thereby reducing swelling of the throat. Epinephrine acts on the beta-1 adrenergic receptors in the heart to increase contractility and heart rate leading to an increase in cardiac output for the maintenance of blood pressure. Additionally, it also exhibits beta-2 adrenergic activity which leads to bronchodilation.

## Steroids

*For more information on steroids and their visual mnemonics, see steroids section (page 35).*

***Steroids*** can help reverse this life-threatening situation. Steroids may be administered when a single dose of epinephrine is ineffective as they suppress the immune system and prevent the release of mediators that are linked with the allergic response.

## Antihistamines

*For more information on antihistamines and their visual mnemonics, see antihistamines section (page 7).*

***Antihistamines*** also serve as a second-line therapy for the treatment of anaphylaxis. In a life-threatening situation antihistamines are administered intravenously to ensure the therapeutic dose reaches the bloodstream in the shortest period of time. In milder cases of anaphylaxis, antihistamines can be administered orally or intramuscularly.

## Inhalers/Nebulizers

For patients who are wheezing, ***inhalers*** and ***nebulizers*** containing bronchodilators can be administered to counteract bronchospasms.

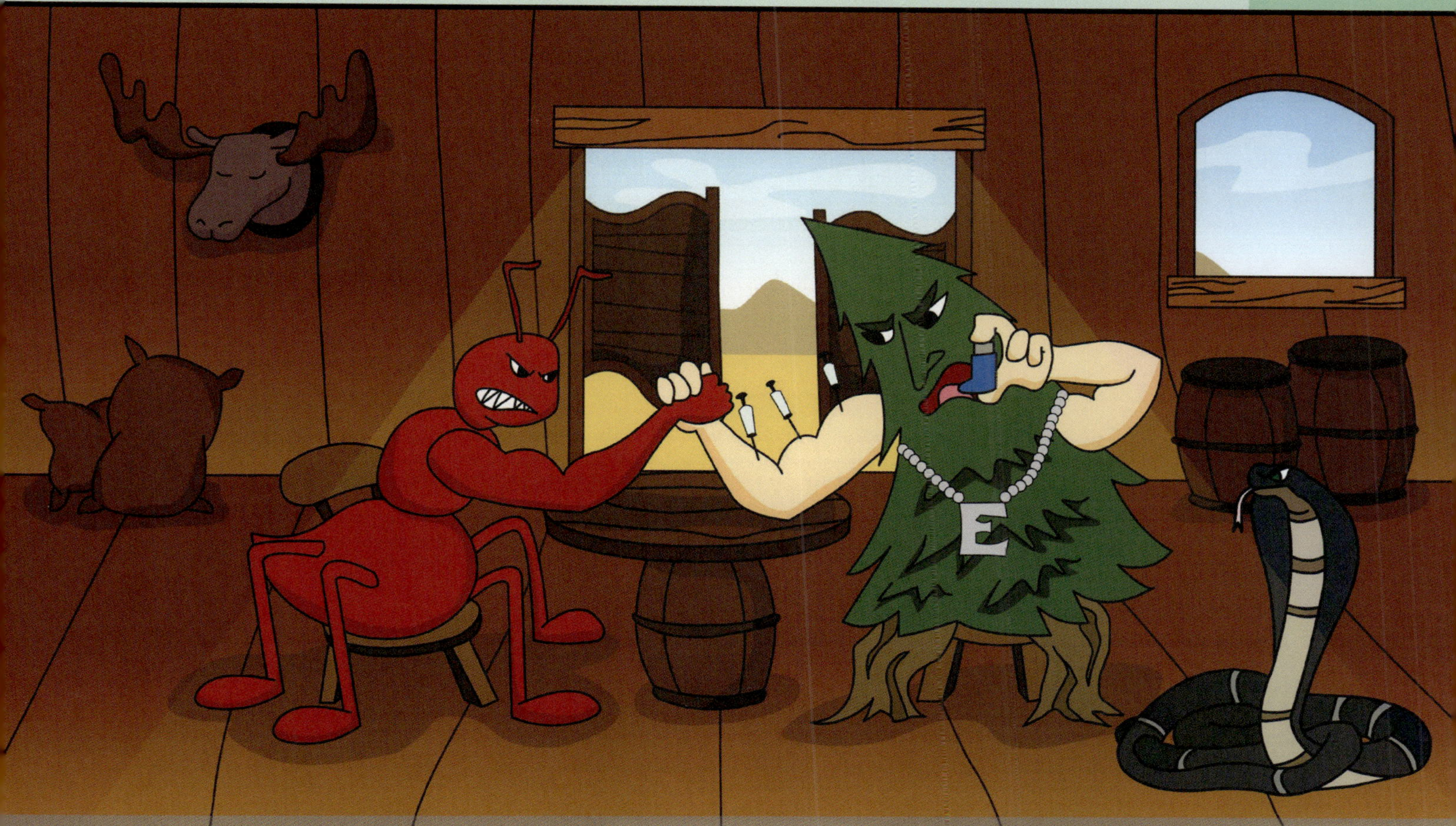

*How to beat anaphylaxis!*

## ANAPHYLAXIS MEDICATIONS

*The ant-flexing reminds you this picture is about anaphylaxis!*

### Epinephrine

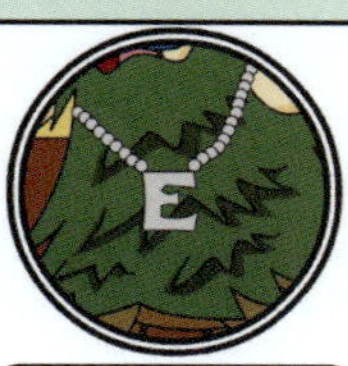

*"E-Pine"*
**Epinephrine**

### Steroids

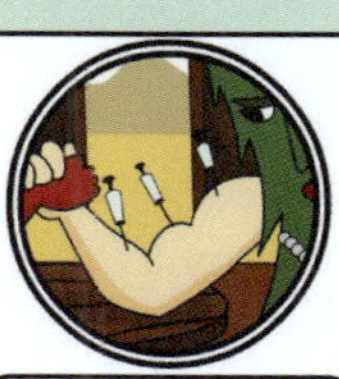

*"Steroids"*
**Steroids**

### Antihistamines

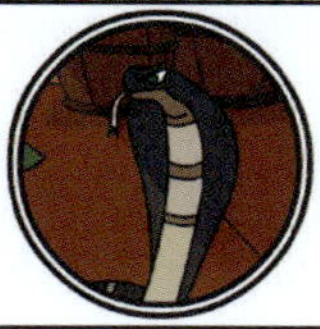

*"Hssssss"*
**Antihistamines**

### Inhalers/Nebulizers

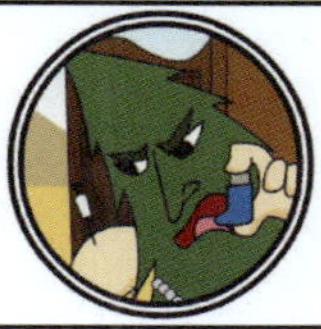

*"Inhalers"*
**Inhalers/nebulizers**

# NSAIDS & ACETAMINOPHEN

**Indications for NSAIDs:** pyrexia, headaches/migraines, gout, musculoskeletal pain (e.g. joint, bone).

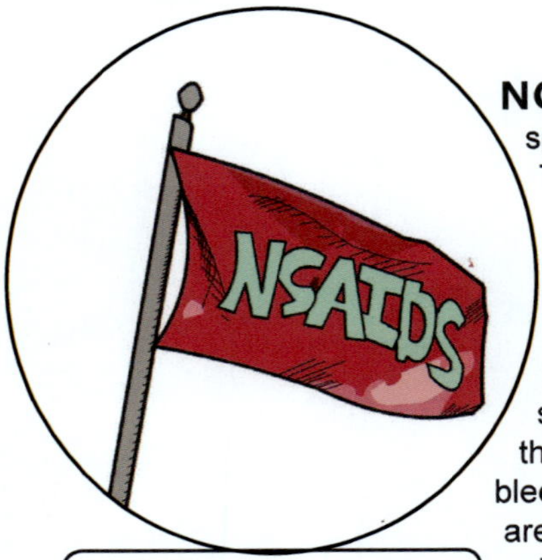


The "NSAID" flag reminds you this picture is about NSAIDS.

**NONSTEROIDAL ANTI-INFLAMMATORY DRUGS (NSAIDS)** have a wide spectrum of activity which include analgesic, anti-pyretic, and anti-inflammatory effects. They can be classified according to their chemical structures and mechanisms of action.

NSAIDs assert their actions by blocking the effects of an enzyme called cyclooxygenase-1 (COX-1) and/or cyclooxygenase-2 (COX-2) which catalyse the formation of prostaglandins and thromboxanes from arachidonic acid. Prostaglandins and thromboxanes play a role in platelet aggregation, vascular tone, and help protect the stomach mucosa from its acidic environment. Subsequently, side effects from blocking these enzymes can cause stomach pain and heartburn, stomach ulcers, a tendency to bleed more, and kidney and liver problems. To reduce the risk of gastric bleeding, NSAIDs are often taken in combination with proton pump inhibitors such as omeprazole to reduce the acidity of the stomach.

## NSAIDs: Irreversible: Aspirin

Like most NSAIDs, ***aspirin*** non-selectively blocks COX enzymes, however, unlike other NSAIDs, it does so irreversibly, allowing aspirin to help with long-term inhibition of blood platelet aggregation. It is an important part of treatment for those with myocardial infarction and stroke, with studies showing that its use leads to a decrease in mortality. Other diseases that warrant the use of aspirin include Kawasaki disease, rheumatic fever, pericarditis, gout, and chronic inflammatory diseases (such as rheumatoid arthritis).

## NSAIDs: Reversibile

### Propionic Acid Derivatives: *Ibuprofen* and *Naproxen*

Another class of NSAIDs comes from propionic acid derivatives, examples include ***ibuprofen*** and ***naproxen***. These two drugs are reversible nonselective COX-inhibitors, where they inhibit both COX-1 and COX-2. Ibuprofen is often used to provide symptom relief in mild to moderate pain conditions such as headache, joint pain and/or fever. Since ibuprofen is nephrotoxic and hepatotoxic, it should not be used in patients who have kidney or liver function impairment.

### Acetic Acid Derivatives: *Diclofenac* and *Indomethacin*

Acetic acid derivatives such as ***diclofenac*** and ***indomethacin*** are also classified as reversible NSAIDs. The use of diclofenac is mainly for the treatment of chronic inflammatory joint disorders such as rheumatoid arthritis, spondyloarthritis, and ankylosing spondylitis. It can also be used to treat colicky pain caused by gallstone or kidney stone impaction.

### Anthranilic Acid Derivatives: *Mefenamic acid*

***Mefenamic acid*** is used in pain associated with gynaecological disorders such as menorrhagia. Its mechanism of action is similar to other types of NSAIDs where they inhibit both COX-1 and COX-2. However, mefenamic acid works particularly well to loosen muscles of the uterus and relieve pain. Adverse effects of mefenamic acid include nausea, vomiting, and diarrhoea. In more severe cases it may lead to blood in the urine or haematemesis.

### COX-2 Selective: *Celecoxib*

***Celecoxib*** is a COX-2 selective NSAID and is commonly used for the treatment of osteoarthritis, rheumatoid arthritis, muscle pain, and/or pain associated with menstruation. The adverse effects are similar to other NSAIDs.

## Miscellaneous Analgesics: Acetaminophen

Finally, ***acetaminophen*** is not an NSAID but acts in a similar fashion. The main difference is that acetaminophen does not exhibit anti-inflammatory effects, therefore, it is used mainly for the relief of fever and pain. Acetaminophen has a good safety profile but in extremely high doses can lead to liver toxicity.

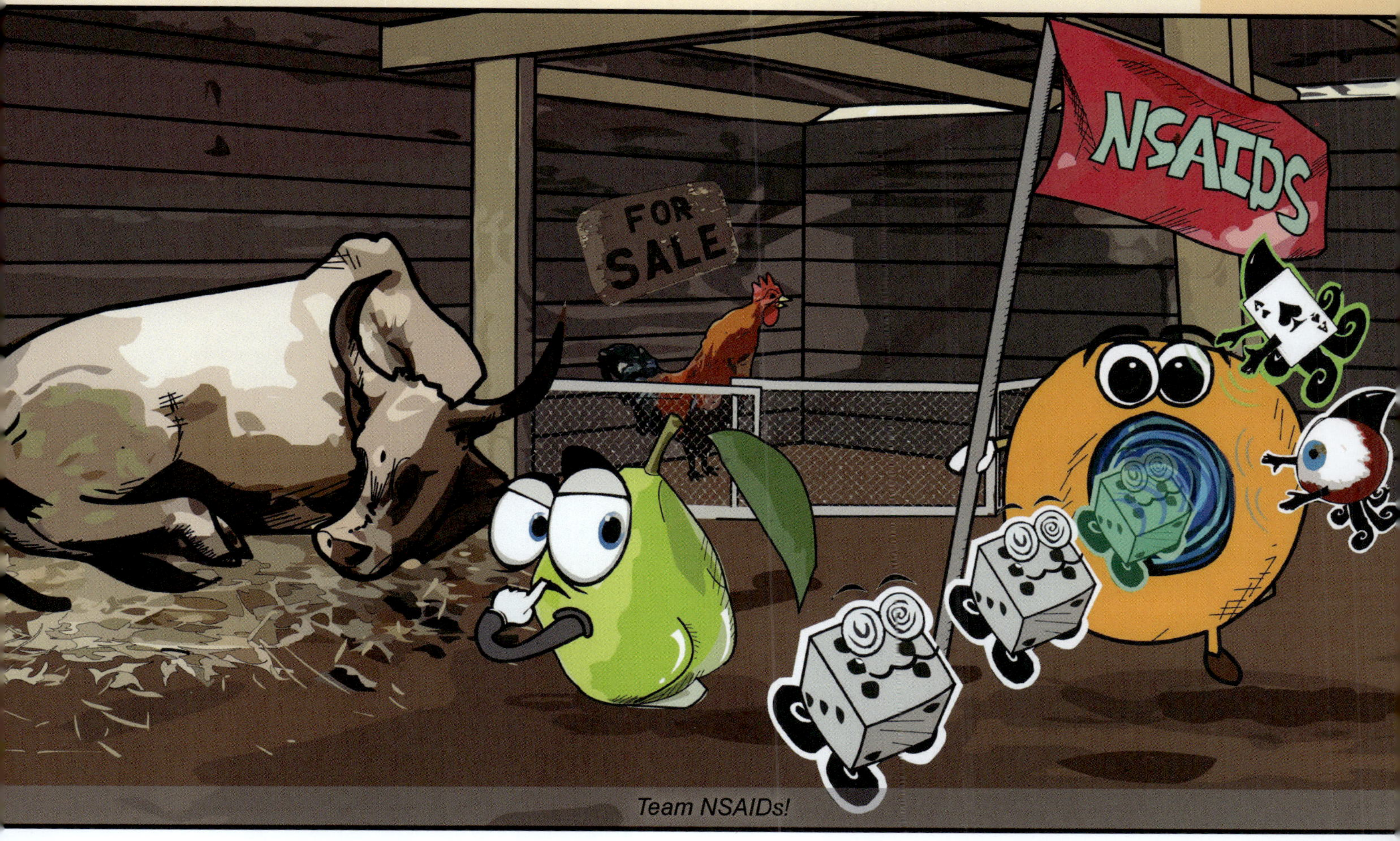

Team NSAIDs!

## NON-STEROIDAL ANTI-INFLAMMATORY DRUGS (NSAIDS)

*The "NSAID" flag reminds you this picture is about NSAIDS*

### NSAIDs

#### Irreversible

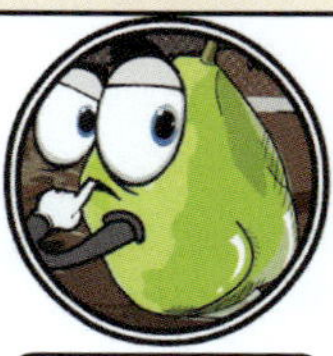

*"Ass-Pear"*
**Aspirin**

#### Reversible

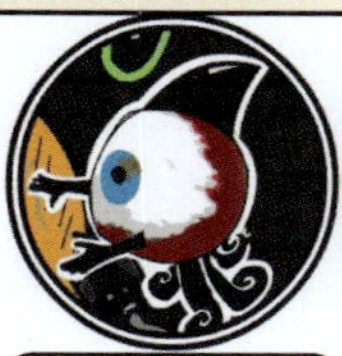

*"Eye-Fin"*
**Ibuprofen**

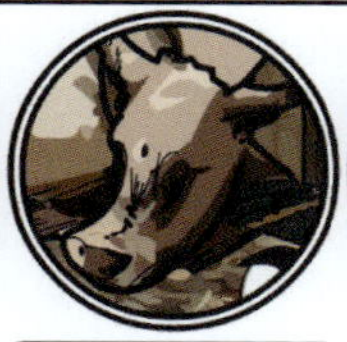

*"Napping-Ox"*
**Naproxen**

PROPIONIC ACID

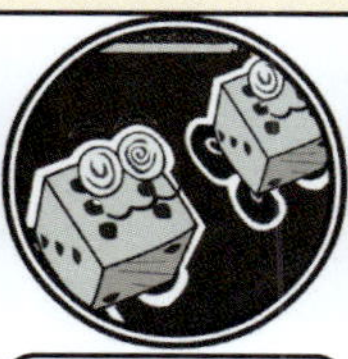

*"Dice-Clone"*
**Diclofenac**

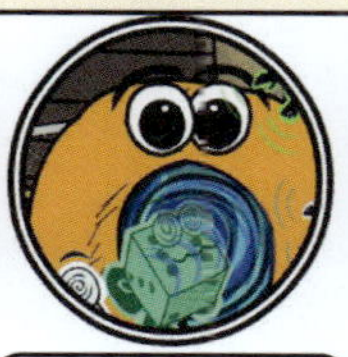

*"In-Donut"*
**Indomethacin**

ACETIC ACID

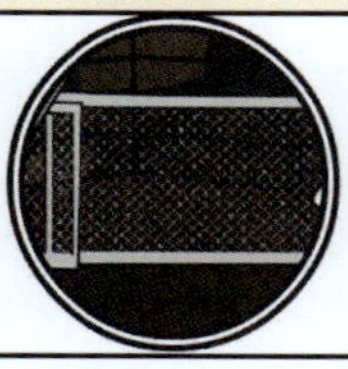

*"Metal-Fence"*
**Mefenamic Acid**

Anthranilic

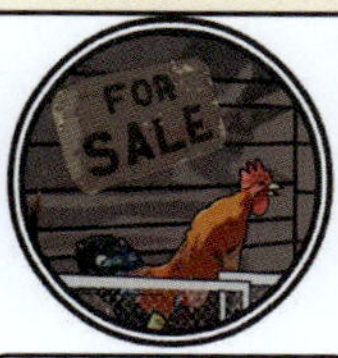


*"Sell-A-Cock"*
**Celecoxib**

COX-2

### MISCELLANEOUS ANALGESICS (not NSAIDs)

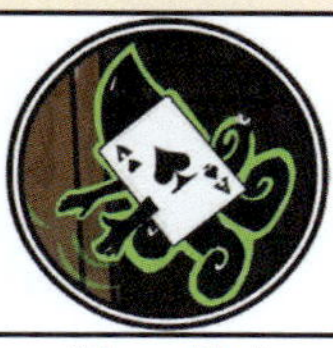

*"Ace-Fin"*
**Acetaminophen**

# OPIOID ANALGESICS

**Indications for opioid analgesics:** pain not controlled with less potent analgesics.

**OPIOIDS** are substances that act as either agonists or antagonists at opioid receptors in the body. They are strictly regulated in many countries due to their high abuse potential. The most common use of opioids are to relieve pain, but they are also used for anesthesia.

Opioids may be natural, semi-synthetic or synthetic, and can be categorized as strong or weak.

Opioids act on three different subtypes of opioid receptors known as the mu, kappa, and delta receptors. Activation of each of these receptors facilitates different physiological actions in the body.

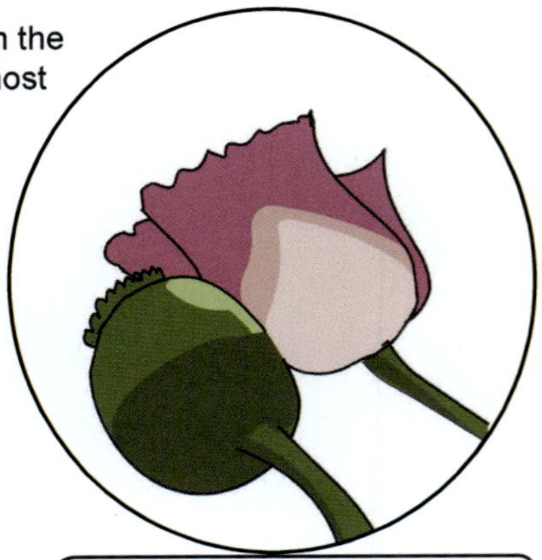

The opioid plants in background remind you this picture is about opioids.

## Opioid Analgesics: Strong Opioids

***Morphine*** is one of the most common drugs used to relieve acute and chronic pain. In the clinical setting, it may be used for the acute management of pain due to myocardial infarction and pain during childbirth. It can be taken through various route of administration including intravenously, intramuscularly, subcutaneously, orally and rectally. Common side effects include hypotension and respiratory depression due to inhibition of the central nervous system.

***Heroin*** is very similar to morphine. It is of higher potency and is created by combining morphine with a reagent called acetic anhydride. Once heroin gets to the brain, it is converted into Morphine and acts upon the same receptors.

***Oxycodone*** is a moderate potent opioid that is also very similar to morphine and acts on the same receptors. It is derived from thebaine and is usually taken in pill form.

***Fentanyl*** is a synthetic opioid that is 50-100 times more potent than morphine, therefore, the dosage must be strictly monitored to prevent toxicity. Fentanyl skin-patches have become popular in management of chronic pain, but it is also used in injectable forms.

***Pethidine*** is a synthetic opioid of the phenylpiperidine class. It acts on the same receptors as morphine and is usually taken orally, intramuscularly, or subcutaneously.

## Opioid Analgesics: Weak Opioids

Weak opioids are often used in combination with NSAIDs to treat mild to moderate pain.

***Codeine*** is an example of a weak opioid. It is commonly used to treat coughs and to relieve diarrhea in irritable bowel syndrome. Common side effects of codeine include drowsiness and constipation.

## Treatment for Opioid Addiction

Consumption of opioids can lead to drug dependence and tolerance. Abrupt discontinuation of this drug can lead to physical and psychological withdrawal symptoms driven by the sympathetic nervous system. As such, there are drugs used as substitutes during rehabilitation therapy to treat withdrawal symptoms.

***Methadone*** is a strong opioid that has been used to treat opioid addiction. It works by acting as an agonist at mu receptors and as an antagonist at NMDA receptors. The exact effect this has in the body is unclear, but the end result is a decrease in craving for opioids, improving withdrawal symptoms, and decreasing tolerance.

***Buprenorphine*** binds to the brain's opioid receptors in place of addictive drugs like morphine and heroin. This produces a reaction in the brain similar to strong opioid agonists, which has the overall effect of improving withdrawal symptoms. It can be used as a second line treatment to prevent nausea/vomiting and to relieve pain in individuals who cannot tolerate first line agents. Common adverse effects of buprenorphine are drowsiness, orthostatic hypotension, urinary retention, and constipation.

## Treatment for Opioid Overdose

***Naloxone*** is administered as treatment in opioid overdose. As naloxone is a pure opioid antagonist, it binds competitively with morphine to mu-receptors to reverse side effects of overdose.

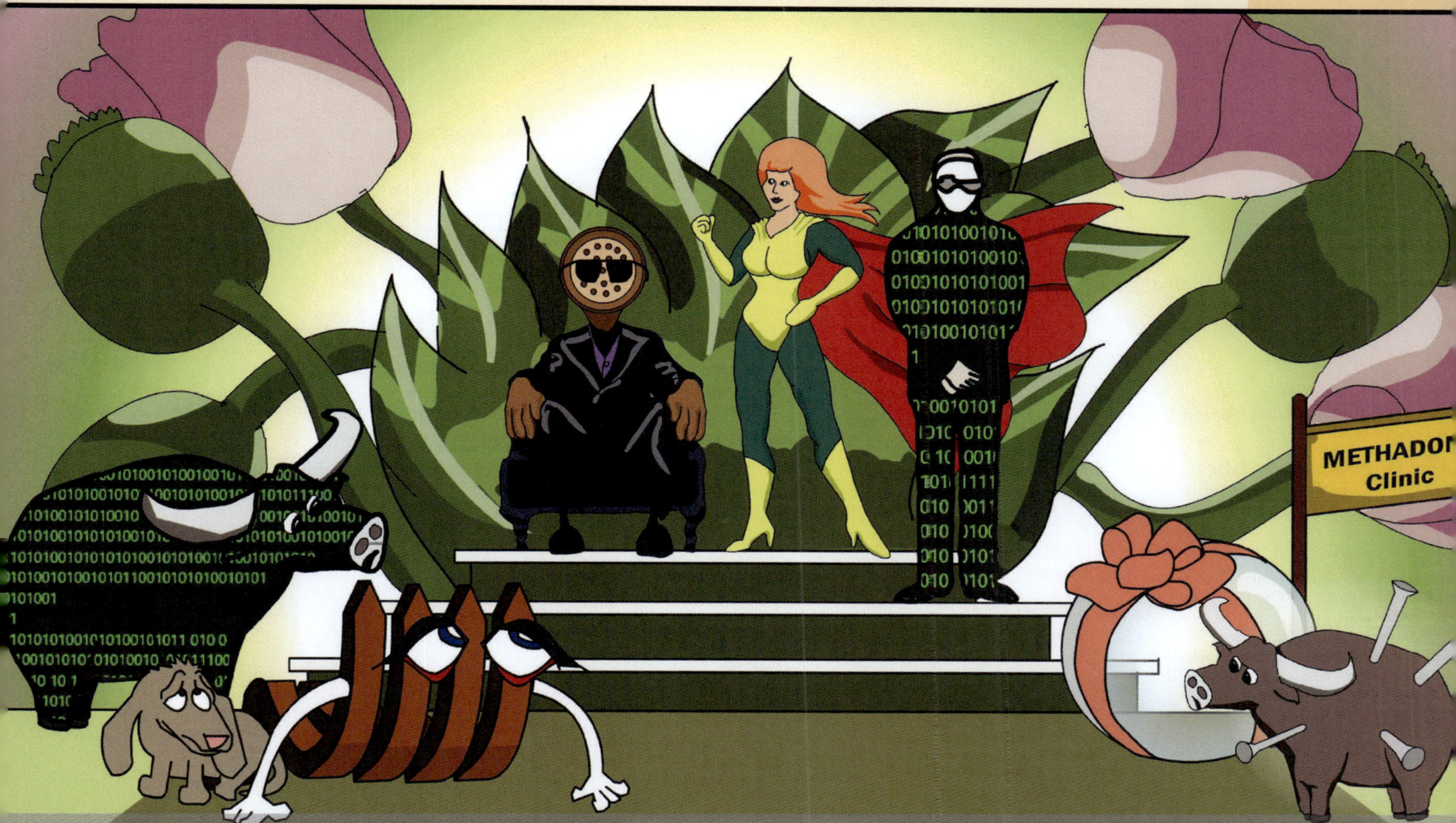


*Team opioid assemble!*

## OPIOID ANALGESICS

☞ *The opioid plants in background remind you this picture is about opioids.*

### Strong Opioids

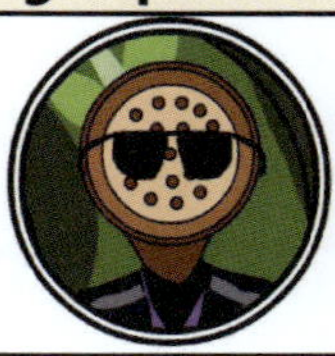

*"Morpheus-Phone"*
**Morphine**

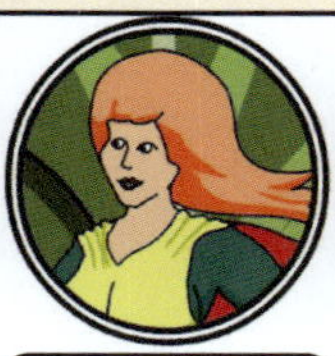

*"Heroine"*
**Heroin**

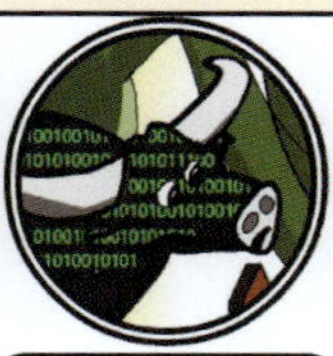

*"Ox-Code"*
**Oxycodone**

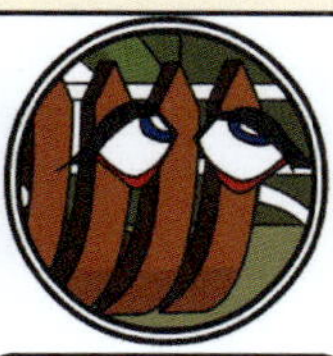

*"Fence-Kneel"*
**Fentanyl**

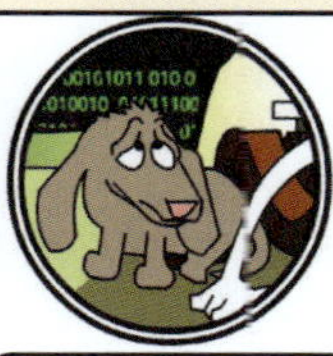

*"Pet-Hiding"*
**Pethidine**

### Weak Opioids

*"Code-Being"*
**Codeine**

### Treatment for Opioid Addiction

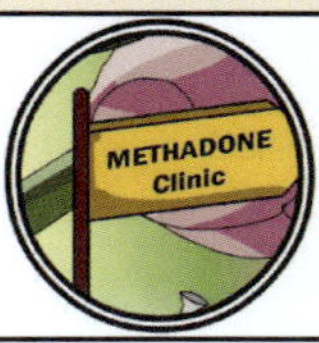


*"Methadone [clinic]"*
**Methadone**

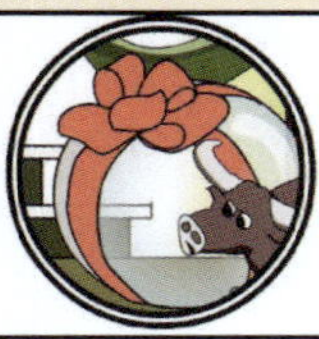

*"Bubble-Present"*
**Buprenorphine**

### Treatment for Opioid Toxicity

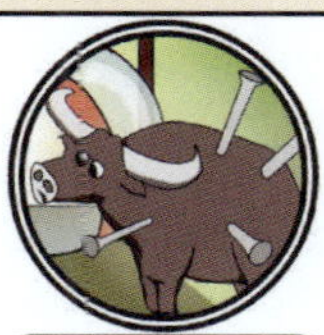

*"Nail-Ox"*
**Naloxone**

# LOCAL ANESTHETICS

**Indications for local anesthetics:** minor procedures (ie. suturing, fracture reduction, excisions).

**LOCAL ANESTHETICS** are a type of medication used to temporarily block pain receptors in nerve cells in a restricted area of the body. Local anesthetics are used mainly for medical and surgical procedures. There are two main classifications of local anesthetics, amides and esters; with each type of anesthetic possessing its own onset of action, duration of effect, and indication.

Both amides and esters aim to stabilize neuron membranes. They bind at sodium voltage-gated channels and prevent the influx of sodium ions through the nerve cell membrane and, as a result, the frequency of action potential firing decreases and the rate of depolarization slows down. When a nerve cell loses the ability to transmit nerve impulses, the patient loses sensation in the region at which the nerve supplies. Amides and esters mainly differ from each other in their chemical structures and properties.

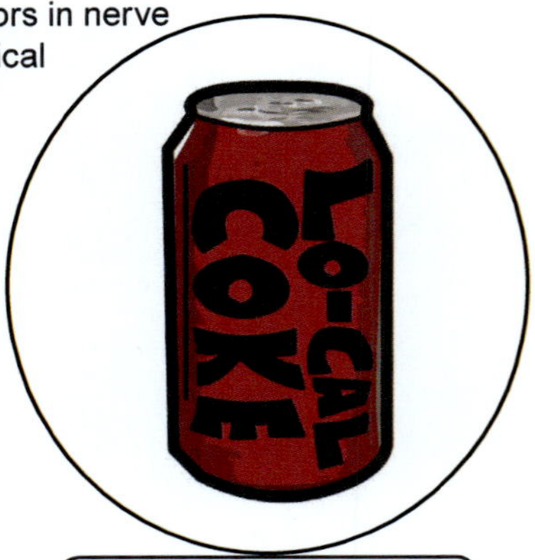


The "Lo-Cal" [low calorie] on the coke bottle, reminds you this picture is about local anesthetics!

## Amides

Examples of amides used in local anesthesia include ***lidocaine, bupivacaine,*** and ***prilocaine***.

***Lidocaine*** has a rapid onset of action and can last up to three hours. It is often used locally to block nerve tissues before minimally invasive procedures. When used in combination with a vasoconstrictor, such as adrenaline, its duration is extended due to delayed resorption.

***Bupivacaine*** has a longer onset of action of approximately fifteen minutes, and it also has a longer duration of effect, up to eight hours. It can be used for peripheral nerve blocks, sympathetic nerve blocks during upper limb surgery, or be applied through the epidural space. Due to its long duration of effect, this drug can be used as an epidural during labor or as a post-operative pain reliever. Bupivacaine is cardiotoxic and should not be administered in patients with heart disease. Rarely, allergic reactions may occur.

***Prilocaine*** is often used in combination with lidocaine in dentistry. Because of its low cardiotoxicity property, prilocaine serves as a good replacement for bupivacaine in patients who have cardiac disease. It is also used in intravenous regional anesthesia, also known as Bier block, an anesthetic procedure carried out before upper limb surgeries.

## Esters

Ester anesthetics include ***cocaine, benzocaine, tetracaine,*** and ***procaine***.

***Cocaine*** is the only naturally occurring local anesthetic, and the first to be used for this purpose. Nowadays, it is rarely used for medical purposes due to its highly addictive nature and stimulation of the cardiovascular system.

***Benzocaine*** is indicated for a wide spectrum of medical conditions including as a pain reliever for mouth ulcers, toothaches, and sore gums. Benzocaine is well-tolerated and has a good safety profile.

***Tetracaine*** is a fast-acting local anesthetic often used to numb the eyes, nose, and throat. Allergic reactions are uncommon.

***Procaine*** is used to decrease pain in medical and dental procedures, but its use has decreased as lidocaine has a lesser chance of allergic reactions.

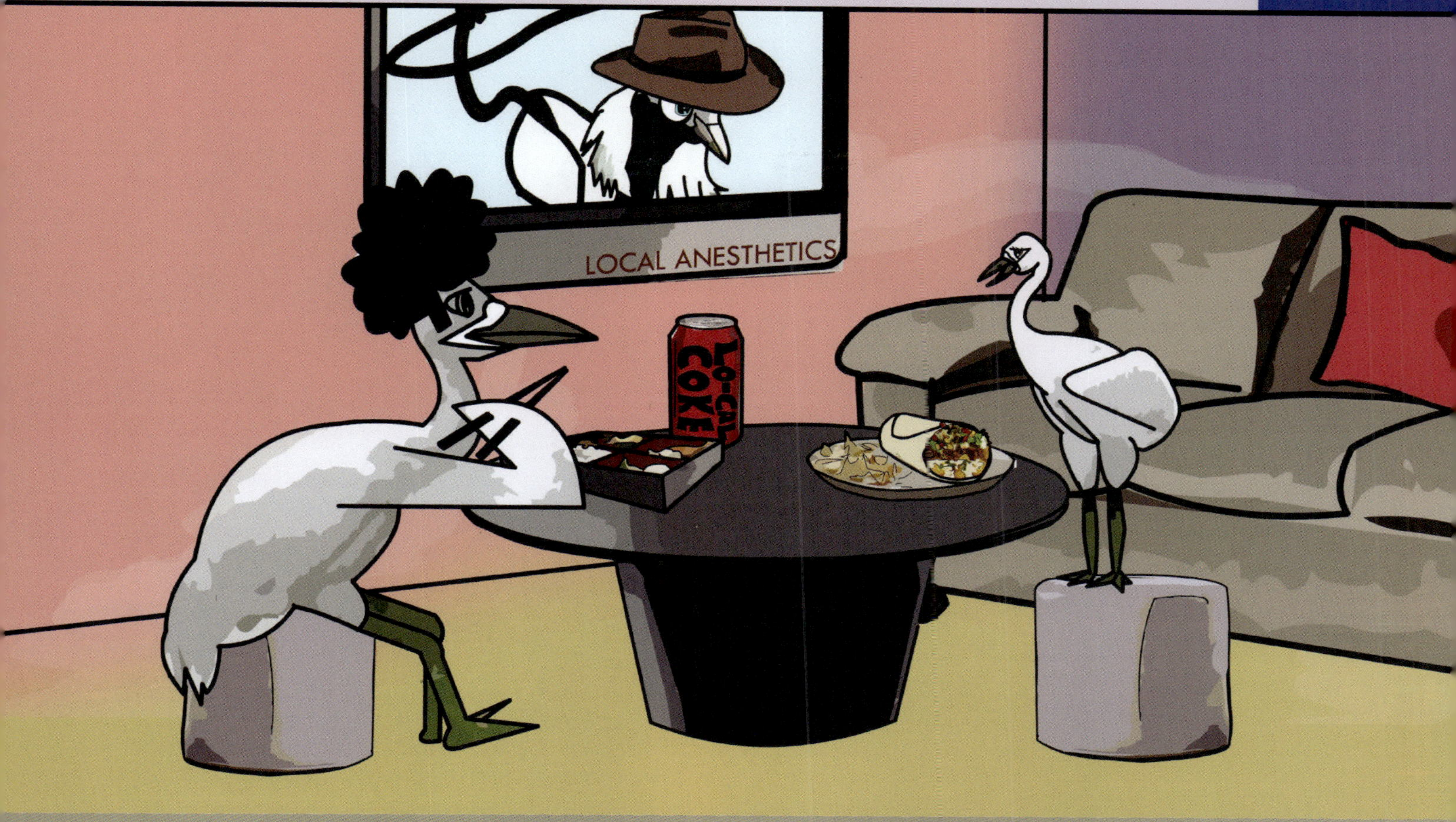


*Just chillin'*

## LOCAL ANESTHETICS

☞ *The "Lo-Cal" [low calorie] on the coke bottle, reminds you this picture is about local anesthetics!*

### Amides

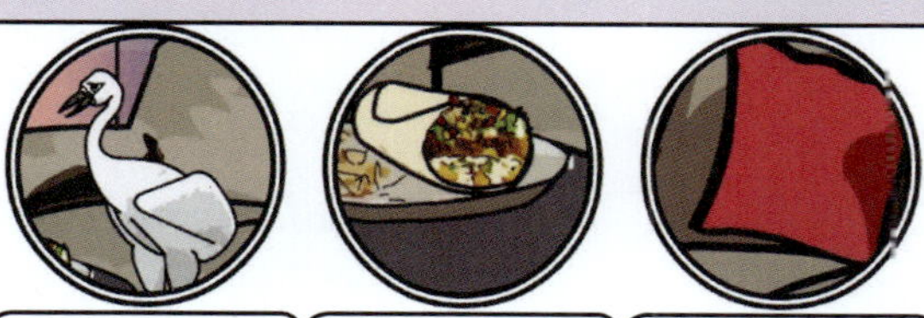

| "Little-Crane" | "Burrito-[Crane]" | "Pillow-[Crane]" |
| --- | --- | --- |
| **Lidocaine** | **Bupivacaine** | **Prilocaine** |

### Esters

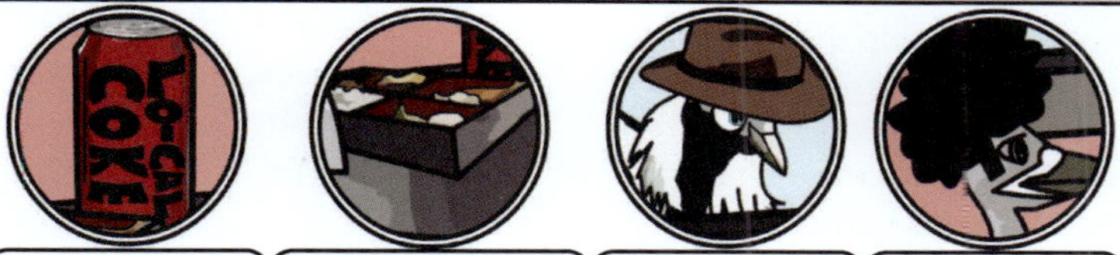

| "Coke-[Crane]" | "Bento-[Crane]" | "Texas-Crane" | "Fro-Crane" |
| --- | --- | --- | --- |
| **Cocaine** | **Benzocaine** | **Tetracaine** | **Procaine** |

# GENERAL ANESTHETICS

**Indications for general anesthetics:** surgical procedures that would be intolerable if conscious.

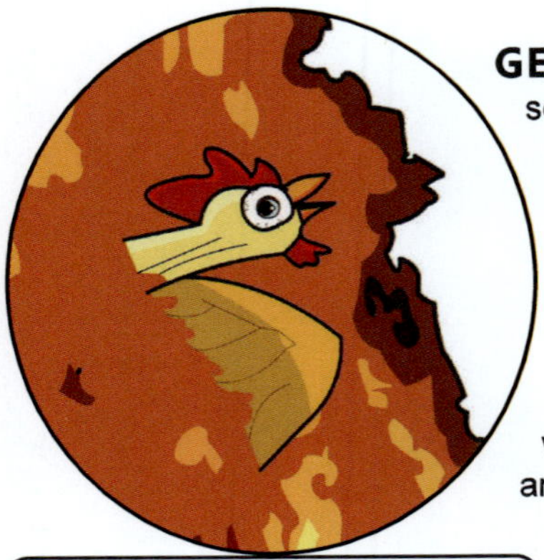

The chicken in this picture could sure use a general anesthetic for the pain!

**GENERAL ANESTHETICS** are drugs which produce a reversible loss of all modalities of sensation and consciousness. These drugs are usually administered by an anesthesiologist in order to induce or maintain a state of general anesthesia during surgical procedures. General anesthetics may be administered either intravenously or through inhalation. The ideal result of general anesthesia comprises of four cardinal features: loss of consciousness, sleep and amnesia, muscle relaxation, and abolition of both somatic and autonomic reflexes.

There are three important phases in general anesthesia. The first phase is induction, which begins from the administration of an anesthetic up to the development of surgical anesthesia. The second phase is the maintenance phase which is defined as the sustaining of the state of anesthesia. Lastly, the recovery phase is where the anesthetics is stopped and the patient begins to regain consciousness.

Pharmacologically, general anesthetics can be classified by the route of administration: ***inhalational*** and ***intravenous***.

## Inhalational Anesthetics

Inhalational anesthetics are responsible for inducing the state of general anesthesia during surgery. The drugs under this category are gases such as ***nitrous oxide*** or volatile liquids like ***halothane***, ***isoflurane***, ***enflurane*** and ***desflurane***. We will discuss two of the more commonly used inhalational anesthetics: nitrous oxide and halothane.

***Nitrous oxide's*** mechanism of action is not fully understood, but it is been shown to modulate a broad range of targets. This includes blocking NMDA receptors, $GABA_C$ receptors and 5-HT3 receptors, and stimulating $GABA_A$ and glycine receptors.

***Halothane*** can be used to start or maintain the state of general anesthesia. Similar to nitrous oxide, it is able to activate $GABA_A$ and glycine receptors and inhibit NMDA receptors in the brain. It is important to note that halothane is capable of triggering a serious complication known as malignant hyperthermia and can also lead to a hypermetabolic state of the skeletal muscles which leads to an increase in oxygen demand.

## Intravenous Anesthetics

Intravenous general anesthetics can be used to induce or maintain anesthesia. Some examples of inducting agents include ***propofol***, ***etomidate***, and ***ketamine***.

***Propofol*** can lead to rapid onset of anesthesia and lead to little accumulation of metabolites. It has antiemetic properties and a moderate risk of myocardial depression.

***Etomidate*** has a favorable cardiac safety profile with little hemodynamic instability, but its disadvantage is that it has no analgesic properties, and prolonged usage may result in adrenal suppression.

***Ketamine*** may be used for induction of anesthesia. It has moderate to strong analgesic properties and produces little myocardial depression, making it a suitable agent for anesthesia in those who are hemodynamically unstable. The drawback of using ketamine is that it can induce a state of dissociation.

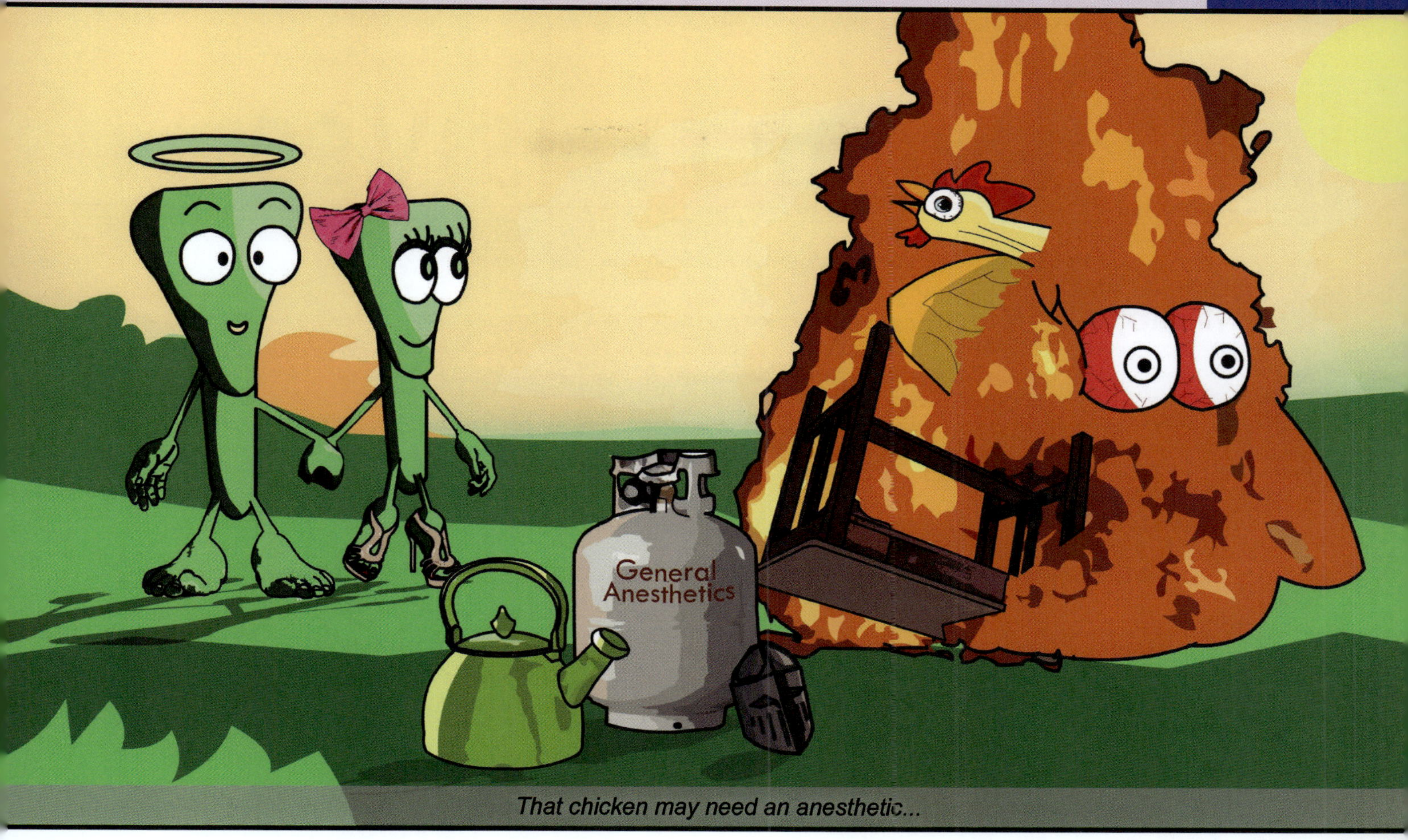


## GENERAL ANESTHETICS

👉 *The chicken in this picture could sure use a general anesthetic for the pain!*

Flam = flurane

### Inhalational

| 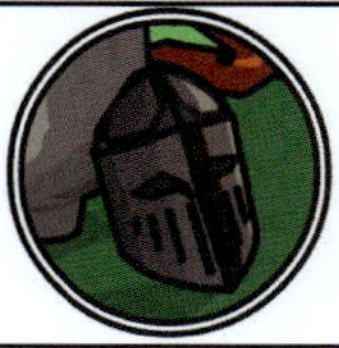 | 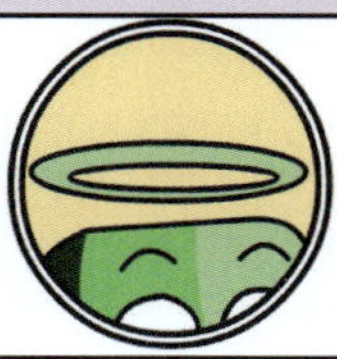 | 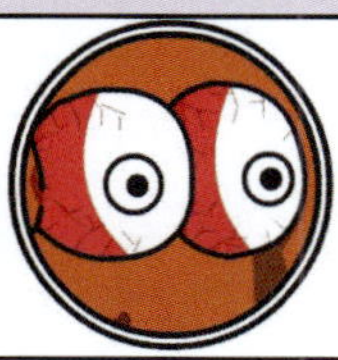 | 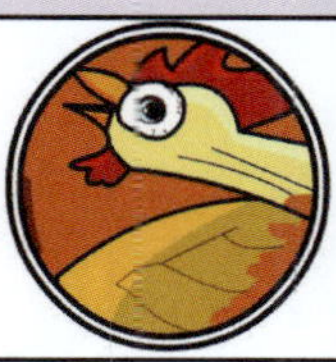 | 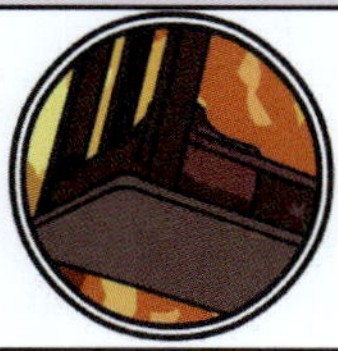 |
|---|---|---|---|---|
| *"Knight-Outside"* **Nitrous Oxide** | *"Halo"* **Halothane** | *"Eye-Flame"* **Isoflurane** | *"Hen-Flame"* **Enflurane** | *"Desk-Flame"* **Desflurane** |

### Intravenous

| 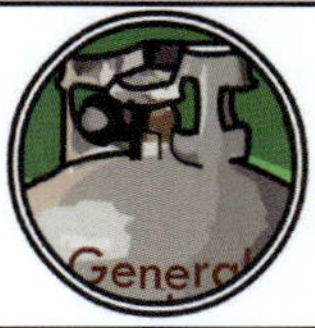 | 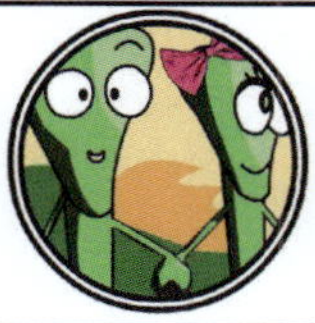 | 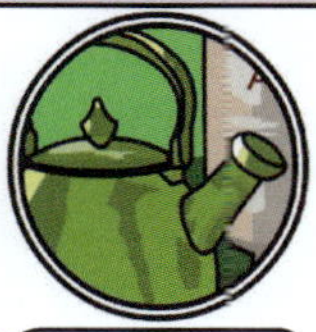 |
|---|---|---|
| *"Propane"* **Propofol** | *"ET-on-date"* **Etomidate** | *"Kettle"* **Ketamine** |

👉 *ET for "Extra-Terrestrial".*

# ANTIHYPERTENSIVES

**Indications for antihypertensive medications:** hypertension.

**HYPERTENSION** is defined as a abnormally high blood pressure, and is clinically measured as resting blood pressure consistently at or above 140/90. Patients with hypertension are frequently asymptomatic until later in disease progression when target organs are affected, when physical activity intolerance, dizziness, headache, palpitations or chest discomfort may occur. Primary hypertension is usually due to unknown etiology, while secondary hypertension is due to a specific cause. The overall goal for the treatment of hypertension is to control the elevated blood pressure and reduce the risk of end organ complications.

## ACE Inhibitors

The initial drug of choice for the treatment of hypertension are angiotensin converting enzyme inhibitors (ACE inhibitors), which prevent the conversion of the peptide hormone angiotensin I to angiotensin II. Angiotensin II facilitates vasoconstriction and therefore, a high systolic pressure is needed to overcome the peripheral resistance. In addition, this peptide hormone also promotes the synthesis of aldosterone, which is a hormone responsible for water and salt reabsorption in the distal convoluted tubules (DCT) and collecting ducts of the kidney nephron; leading to higher blood volume and increased blood pressure. Examples of ACE-inhibitors are ***ramipril***, ***lisinopril*** and ***perindopril***. Side effects include dry cough, hyperkalemia, and fatigue.

## Angiotensin Receptor Blockers (ARBs)

ARBs lower blood pressure by competitively blocking the Angiotensin II receptors thereby preventing vasoconstriction and the synthesis of aldosterone. Examples of ARB's are ***losartan***, ***valsartan***, and ***candesartan***. Side effects of ARB's include hypotension, hyperkalemia and teratogenicity.

## Thiazide Diuretics

Thiazide diuretics act in the DCT of the kidney, where its primary mechanism of action is the inhibition of the sodium chloride symporter, causing the ions in the DCT to be excreted out of the body via urine. These diuretics are usually taken orally and its onset of action is approximately one hour. The side effects of thiazides include hypokalemia, hyponatremia, hyperuricemia, elevated plasma lipids, and diminished insulin secretion. Examples of the thiazide diuretics include ***bendroflumethiazide*** and ***hydrochlorothiazide***.

## Loop Diuretics

Loop diuretics are also used in treating hypertension. These medications inhibit apical sodium-potassium-chloride (Na+K+2Cl-) transporters located in the ascending loop of Henle. This creates a low interstitial osmolality in the nephron, prevents the reabsorption of water, and increases urine production. Loop diuretics such as ***furosemide*** have rapid onset of action. Side effects include hyperuricemia, hypokalemia, metabolic alkalosis and ototoxicity in some cases.

## Calcium Channel Blockers (CCBs)

***Nifedipine*** and ***amlodipine*** are classified as 1,4-dihydropyridines calcium channel blockers. They act by prolonging the closure time of calcium channels. This leads to relaxation of arterial smooth muscle followed by peripheral vasodilation. The outcome of this mechanism is a significant reduction of afterload in the heart. Calcium channel blockers may lead to hypotension, headache and peripheral edema due to fluid accumulation in the lower extremities.

## Beta-Blockers

Beta-blockers play significant role in controlling elevated blood pressure. All beta-blockers have similar antihypertensive effects irrespective of their additional properties from binding various receptors at different locations. They are able to decrease heart rate and lower blood pressure by binding to beta-1 receptors in the heart. Furthermore, they decrease the release of renin from the kidney and reduce sympathetic outflow mediated by catecholamines. Examples include ***metoprolol*** and ***atenolol***.

## Alpha-Blockers

***Prazosin*** and ***doxazosin*** are alpha-1 receptor blockers that act in the arterial vessel wall. By blocking alpha-1 receptors, they inhibit peripheral vasoconstriction and lead to a decrease in afterload. This medication is typically used for treatment of symptoms brought about by benign prostatic hyperplasia, but can be used as a second line treatment in hypertension.

## Centrally Acting Drugs

Centrally acting drugs such as ***methyldopa*** are used to treat hypertension in pregnant patients. It is a competitive inhibitor of an enzyme called DOPA decarboxylase which is responsible for the synthesis of catecholamine and dopamine.

## Vasodilators

Finally, vasodilators such as ***hydralazine*** can also be used to treat hypertension. They bind to the endothelium arteriole receptors and facilitates the release of nitric oxide which leads to smooth muscle relaxation. As a result, blood pressure decreases. Hydralazine may lead to side effects like reflex tachycardia and activation of RAAS system.

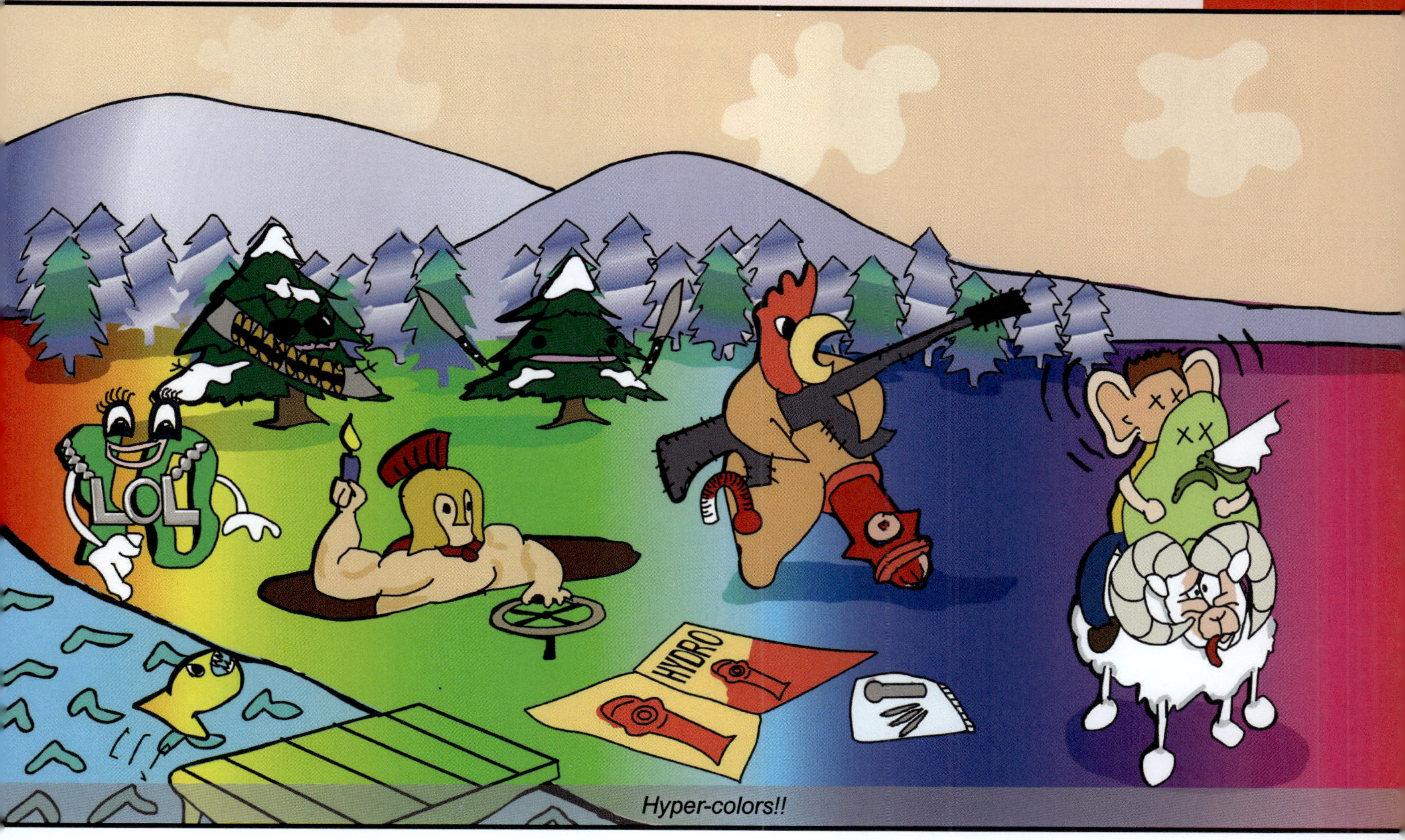

Hyper-colors!!

## HYPERTENSION

The "*hyper*"-colors remind you this picture is about anti-*hyper*tensives.

### ACE Inhibitors

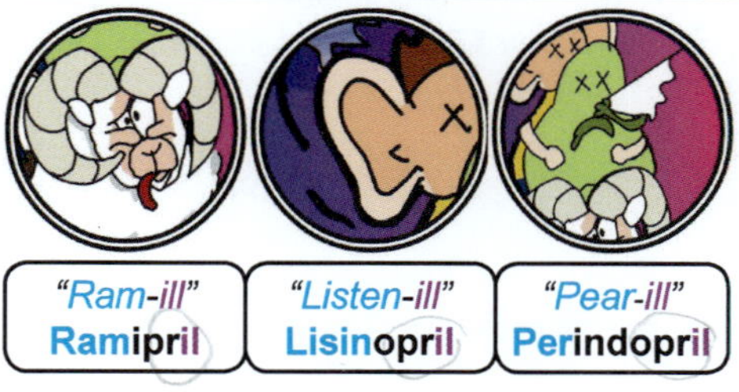

- *"Ram-ill"* **Ramipril**
- *"Listen-ill"* **Lisinopril**
- *"Pear-ill"* **Perindopril**

### ARBs

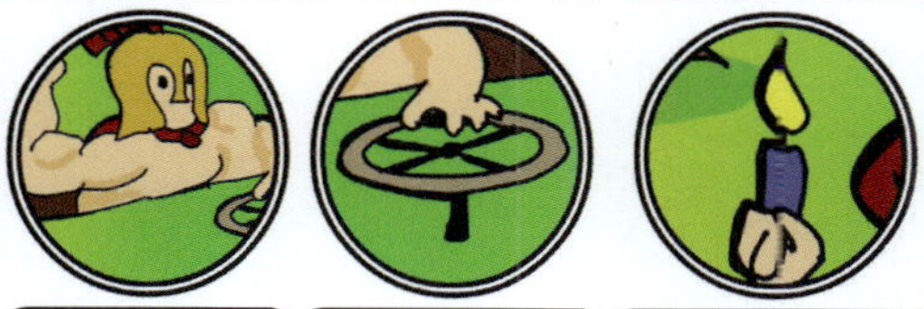

- *"Low-Spartan"* **Losartan**
- *"Valve-Spartan"* **Valsartan**
- *"Candle-Spartan"* **Candesartan**

### Thiazide D.

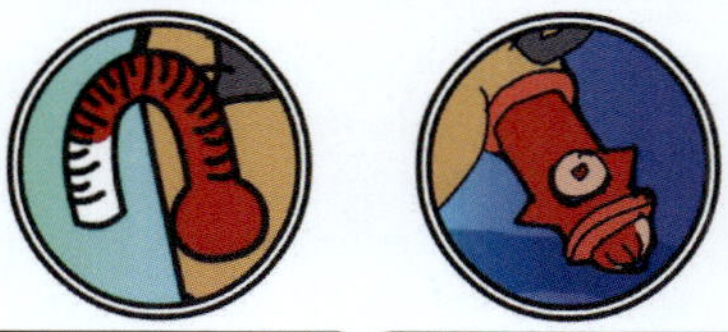

- *"Bend-Flu-Thigh"* **Bendroflumethiazide**
- *"Hydro-Thigh"* **Hydrochlorothiazide**

### Loop D.

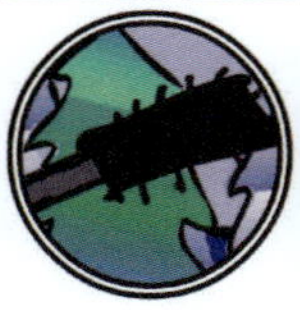

- *"Fur-Semi"* **Furosemide**

### CCBs

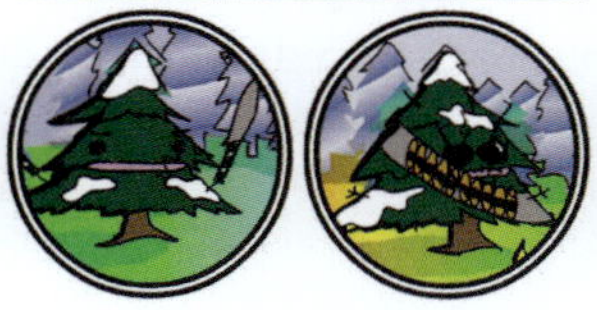

- *"Knife-Pine"* **Nifedipine**
- *"Ammo-Pine"* **Amlodipine**

### Beta-Blockers

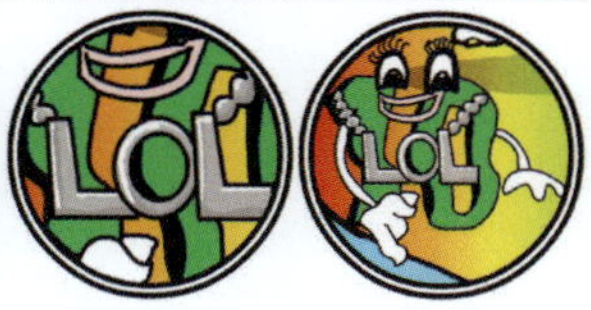

- *"Metal-LOL"* **Metoprolol**
- *"A-Ten-LOL"* **Atenolol**

### Alpha-Blockers

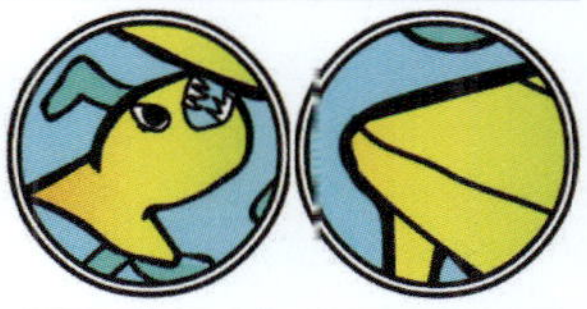

- *"Piranha"* **Prazosin**
- *"Dock"* **Doxazosin**

### Centrally Acting

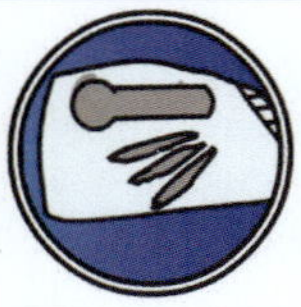

- *"Meth-Dope"* **Methyldopa**

### Others

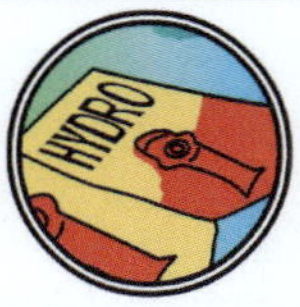

- *"Hydro-Magazine"* **Hydralazine**

# ANTIARRHYTHMICS CLASS I

**Indications for antiarrhythmics:** atrial fibrillation, atrial flutter, ventricular tachycardia, ventricular fibrillation.

**ANTIARRHYTHMICS** are used for the treatment of abnormal electrical impulse conduction in the heart known as arrhythmias. Cardiac arrhythmia may arise in isolation, spontaneously, or it may co-exist with other cardiac diseases.

Arrhythmia is defined as the condition in which the heart beats in an irregular or abnormal rhythm. The heart usually contracts regularly at the rate between 60 to 100 beats per minute. Each heart beat should be originated from the sinoatrial (SA) node and each cardiac impulse should propagate through the conduction pathway with a normal conduction velocity.

Generally, the impulse conduction begins from the wall situated adjacent to the right atrium of the heart in the sinoatrial node (SAN). The main process that takes place in the SAN is depolarization. Depolarization takes place when the threshold for the next electrical impulse conduction is exceeded. This leads to sodium channels opening followed by sodium ions influx. Electrical impulses travel down to the ventricles passing through the atrioventricular node (AVN) before repolarization occurs.

When the impulse conduction pathway gets disrupted, the heart will not be able to pump blood efficiently and will contract in a chaotic manner. In this case, antiarrhythmic drugs have to be administered to control the rhythmicity of the heart.

There are five different classes of antiarrhythmics, each class has different actions which affect the rhythm of the heart uniquely. In this chapter, we will cover antiarrhythmics class I.

## Class I Antiarrhythmics

The class I antiarrhythmics are also called ***sodium channel blockers.***

Class I is sub-classified into three categories: ***IA, IB*** and ***IC***, each differing in their effect on action potential duration and conduction velocity.

## Class IA

Class IA drugs block sodium channels; cause a decrease in the conduction velocity through the heart; and prolongs action potential duration. These drugs act on both the atria and ventricles and can be administered orally or intravenously. They are used in the treatment of atrial fibrillation, re-entrant tachycardia, ventricular tachycardia, and in some cases, in the treatment of a life-threatening form of ventricular tachycardia called torsades-de-pointes.

Examples of class IA antiarrhythmics include ***disopyramide, quinidine*** and ***procainamide***. Quinidine should be noted that its toxicity can cause conditions like cinchonism (headache, tinnitus, vertigo).

## Class IB

Class IB antiarrhythmics have a weaker sodium channel blockade effect than class IA, and therefore cause less of a rise in phase 0 of the ventricular action potential curve and also decreases the effective refractory period. These effects lead to no significant change in the conduction velocity and overall shortened action potential duration.

Usually this class of antiarrhythmics is used to treat ventricular tachycardia to prevent arrhythmias after myocardial infarction. Examples of class IB drugs include ***lidocaine, tocainide,*** and ***mexiletine.***

This class of drug can be used for the treatment of cardiac arrhythmias, and can also be used in other medical conditions. Notably, lidocaine is often used as a local anesthetic. Systemic exposure to lidocaine may lead to functional impairment in the central nervous system (CNS). It can either lead to CNS excitation symptoms such as agitation, hallucination, psychosis, or CNS depression symptoms like drowsiness, slurred speech or respiratory depression.

## Class IC

Class IC antiarrhythmic drugs exhibit strong blocking effects on fast-acting sodium channels, leading to decreased conduction velocity in the heart without a significant effect on action potential duration. Some examples of class IC antiarrhythmic drugs include ***moricizine***, ***flecainide***, and ***propafenone***.

These drugs are suitable to be used to treat supraventricular arrhythmias such as paroxysmal atrial fibrillation, supraventricular tachycardia, and Wolf-Parkinson-White (WPW) syndrome. Similar to other antiarrhythmic drugs, it can lead to proarrhythmia, which is the new occurrence or increasing frequently of pre-existing cardiac arrhythmia.

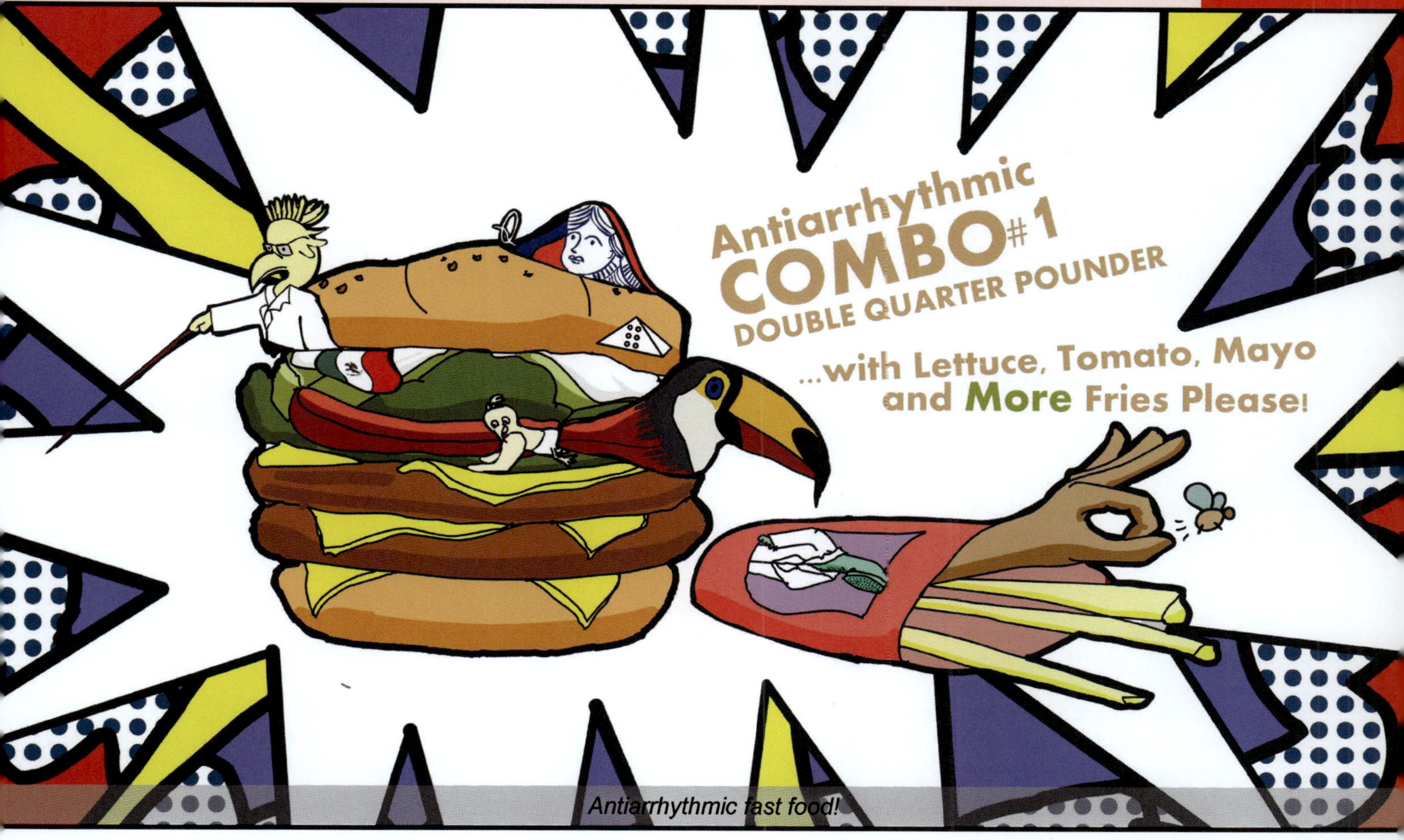

*Antiarrhythmic fast food!*

## CLASS I ANTIARRHYTHMICS: SODIUM CHANNEL BLOCKERS

This picture is a play on the popular word mnemonic **"Double Quarter Pounder, with Lettuce, Tomato, Mayo, and More Fries Please"**. The word mnemonic only helps you remember the first letter of the drug names, our picture will help you remember the full name of each medication.

### Class IA

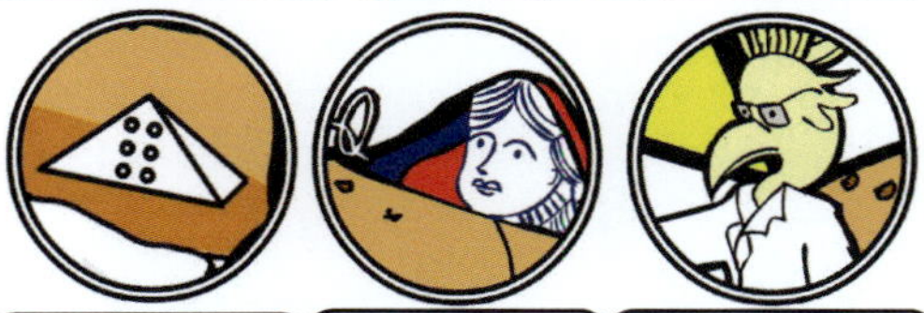

| "Dice" | "Queen" | "Prof-Crane" |
|---|---|---|
| **Disopyramide** | **Quinidine** | **Procainamide** |

### Class IB

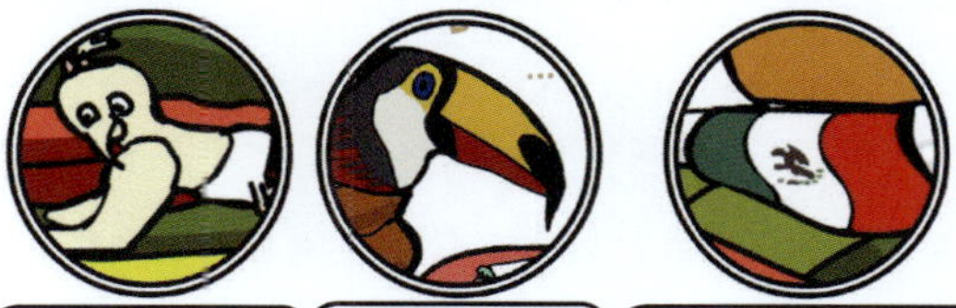

| "Little-Crane" | "Toucan" | "Mexican-Lettuce" |
|---|---|---|
| **Lidocaine** | **Tocainide** | **Mexiletine** |

### Class IC

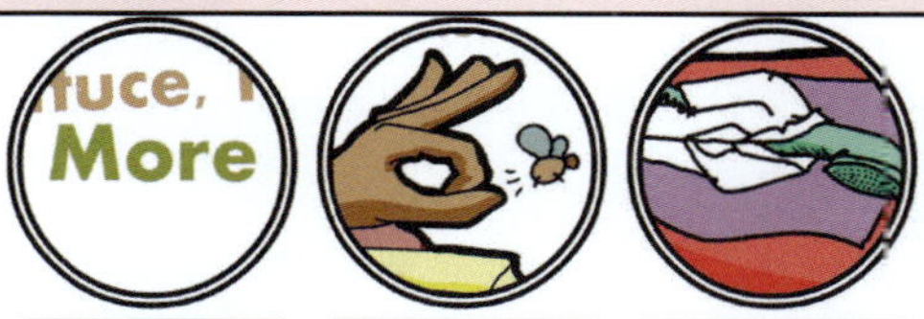


| "More" | "Flick-Fly" | "Prof-Phone" |
|---|---|---|
| **Moricizine** | **Flecainide** | **Propafenone** |

# ANTIARRHYTHMIC CLASS II, III, IV, V

**Indications for antiarrhythmics:** atrial fibrillation, atrial flutter, ventricular tachycardia, ventricular fibrillation.

## AS DISCUSSED IN ANTIARRHYTHMICS CLASS I,

antiarrhythmics are used for the treatment of abnormal electrical impulse conduction in the heart known as arrhythmias.

Antiarrhythmics can be classified as class I, II, III, IV or V. Each category has their own mechanism of action and pharmacological effects, and this section will explore classes II through V.

Both antiarrhythmic pictures are based upon ordering from the "antiarrhythimic" fast food restaurant. Class 2 antiarrhythmics is "Combo #2", class 3 antiarrhythmics is "Combo #3", and so on.

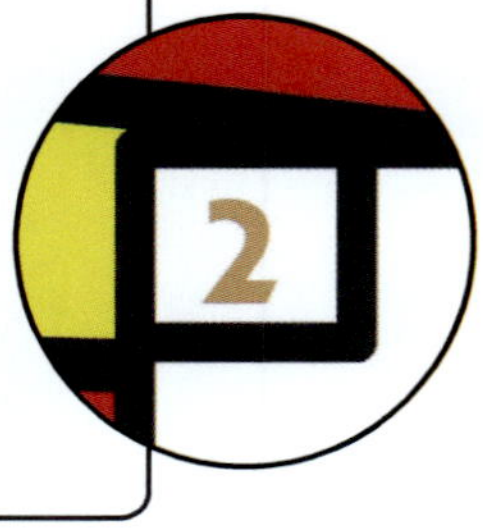


### Class II: Beta-Blockers

The class II antiarrhythmic drugs are known as beta-blockers as they target the beta-adrenergic receptors in the heart. Beta blockers primarily used in cardiovascular disease include ***metoprolol*** and ***atenolol***, which are selective beta-1 receptor antagonists.

The mechanism of these beta-blockers competitively block catecholamine induced stimulation of the cardiac beta-receptors, leading to the depression of phase 4 depolarization of pacemaker cells. As a result, action potential firing from the sinoatrial (SA) node and the atrioventricular (AV) node decreases, and increases the effective refractory period.

Overall, beta-blockers reduce oxygen demand from cardiac muscle tissues and can be used for emergency treatment during atrial flutter, atrial fibrillation, paroxysmal supraventricular tachycardia, ventricular arrhythmias, and in prolonged QT syndrome. They are also used as prophylaxis after myocardial infarction. Beta-blockers may exacerbate asthma and mask signs of hypoglycemia. Toxicity from beta-blockers can be reversed by glucagon.

### Class III: Potassium Channel Blockers

Class III antiarrhythmics are composed of potassium channel blockers such as ***amiodarone*** and ***sotalol***.

***Amiodarone*** is an iodine-containing long-acting drug that blocks potassium channels to prevent the efflux of potassium ions responsible for repolarization. This increases the effective refractory period of cardiac tissues. Amiodarone is indicated for ventricular arrhythmia and as a second line agent during supraventricular arrhythmia. Adverse effects include hypotension, bradycardia and burning sensation at the intravenous site. Amiodarone side effects include pulmonary fibrosis, hepatotoxicity, hypo/hyperthyroidism, and photosensitivity.

Although ***sotalol*** is a beta-blocker, it is considered part of class III as it also acts on potassium channels, leading to a delay in relaxation of ventricles.

### Class IV: Calcium Channel Blockers

Class IV antiarrhythmics are calcium channel blockers such as ***verapamil*** and ***diltiazem***. This class slows spontaneous depolarization in Phase 4 and subsequently slow conduction in tissues dependent on calcium ions such as the AV node.

Ultimately, these work by inhibiting the influx of calcium ions by blocking the calcium channels leading to a decrease in cardiac contractility, automaticity, and AV node conduction. Both these medications can be used to terminate paroxysmal supraventricular tachycardia and control ventricular rate in atrial flutter and atrial fibrillation. Side effects include constipation, dizziness, nausea, and headache.

### Class V: Other

Class V antiarrhythmics are represented by a variety of drugs with other or unknown mechanisms of action. They include ***adenosine***, ***digoxin***, and ***magnesium sulfate***, all of which can be used to manage cardiac arrhythmias.

***Adenosine*** is a purine nucleoside with short and rapid action. It suppresses cardiac automaticity, AV nodal conduction, and dilates coronary arteries. Adenosine is used for diagnosis of supraventricular tachycardia as it provides a transient heart block. Side effects of adenosine include headache, shortness of breath and flushing.

***Digoxin*** can be used in patients with congestive heart failure complicated by atrial fibrillation or atrial flutter. It increases and regulates the heart contractility without affecting the heart rate.

***Magnesium sulfate*** has an unknown mechanism of action, but it is thought to be able to affect sodium-potassium ATPase, potassium channels, and calcium channels. It can be used to treat digoxin-induced arrhythmia, refractory ventricular tachyarrhythmia, and torsade-de-pointes.

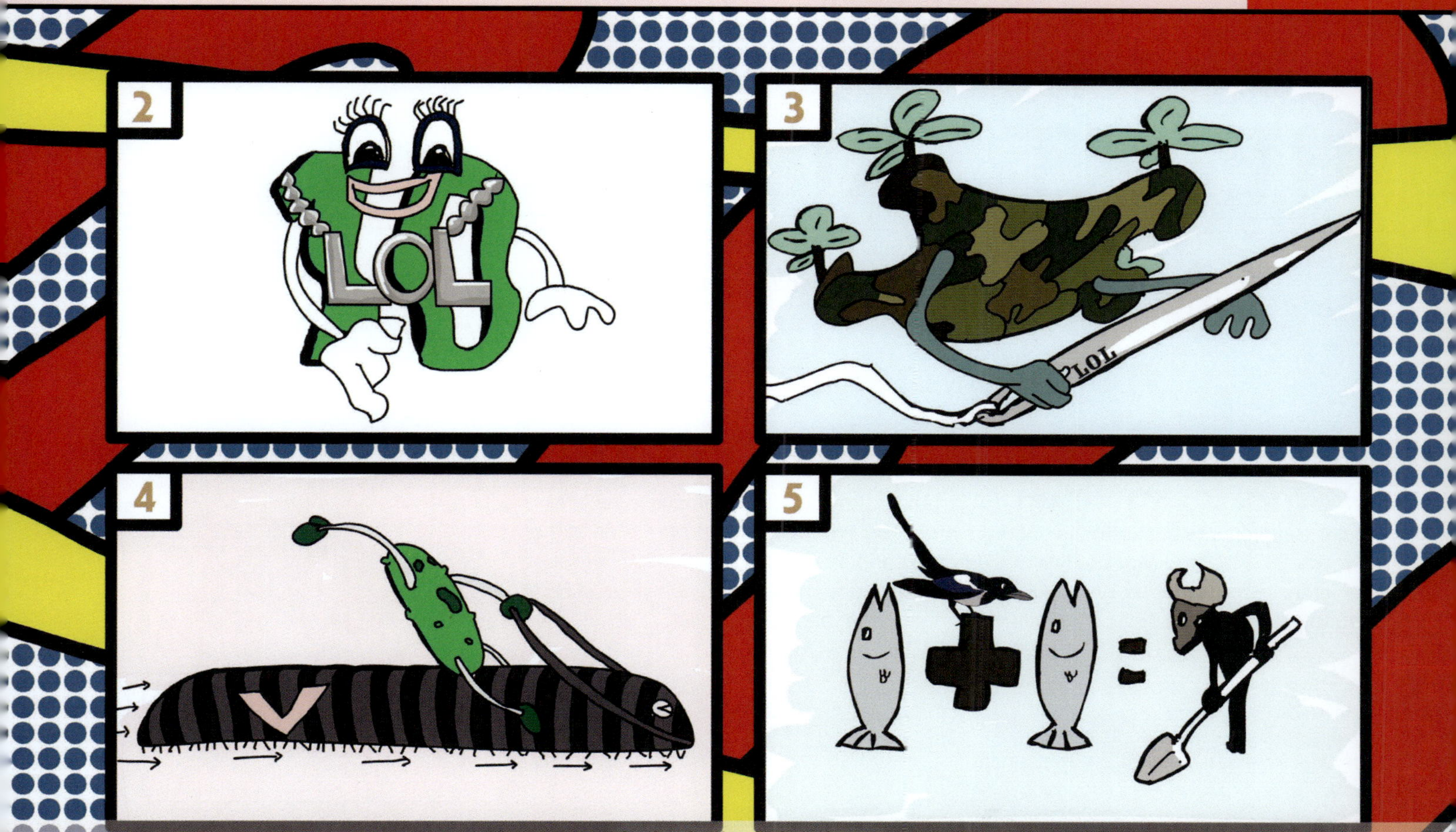


*Antiarrhythmic fast food!*

## ANTIARRHYTHMICS

*Both antiarrhythmic pictures are based upon ordering from the "antiarrhythimic" fast food restaurant. Class 2 antiarrhythmics is "Combo #2", Class 3 antiarrhythmics is "Combo #3", and so on.*

### Class II: Beta-Blockers

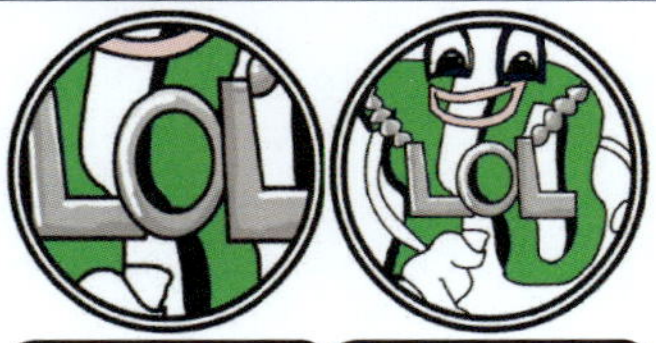

| "Metal-LOL" **Metoprolol** | "A-Ten-LOL" **Atenolol** |
|---|---|

### Class III: Potassium Channel Blockers

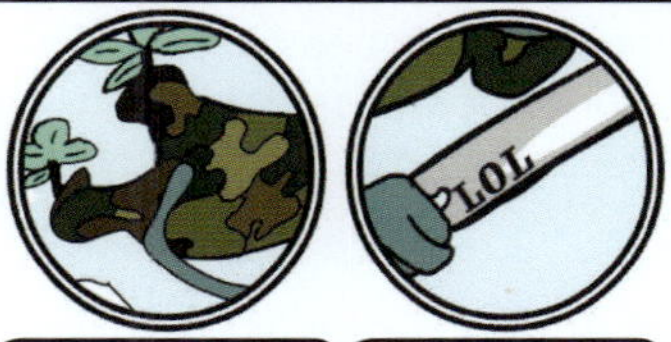

| "Army-Drone" **Amiodarone** | "Sew-LOL" **Sotalol** |
|---|---|

### Class IV: Calcium Channel Blockers

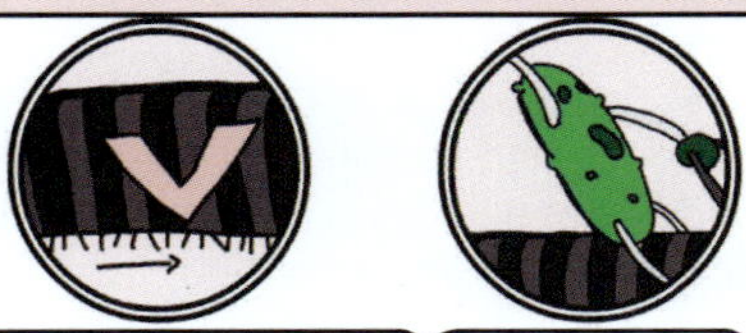

| "Very-[Fast]-Millipede" **Verapamil** | "Dill" **Diltiazem** |
|---|---|

### Class V: Other

| "Add-Sardine" **Adenosine** | "Digg-Ox" **Digoxin** | "Magpie" **Magnesium Sulfate** |
|---|---|---|

# HEART FAILURE

**Indications for heart failure medications:** heart failure.

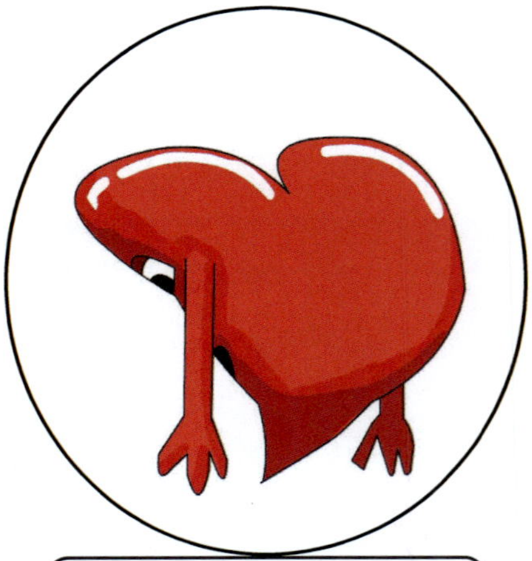

The depressed heart reminds you that this picture is about heart failure!

**IN PATIENTS WITH HEART FAILURE,** the aim of treatment is to relieve major symptoms (e.g. shortness of breath and chest pain) and stop progression of the disease. This is done with lifestyle modifications and medication. Medications include angiotensin converting enzyme (ACE) inhibitors, angiotensin receptor blockers (ARBs), beta-blockers, loop diuretics, aldosterone antagonists, and vasodilators.

## Angiotensin Converting Enzyme (ACE) Inhibitors

ACE inhibitors, such as ***perindopril***, ***lisinopril***, and ***ramipril***; act by inhibiting ACE, an enzyme produced by the endothelial cells in lung capillaries. By blocking ACE, angiotensin I is unable to be converted to angiotensin II, which leads to a downstream inhibition of aldosterone synthesis. Reduced aldosterone levels lead to decreases in salt and water reabsorption in the distal convoluted tubules and collecting ducts of the kidney. The physiological effect is a decrease of blood pressure and cardiac workload. A common side effect of ACE inhibitors is dry cough.

## Angiotensin Receptor Blockers (ARBs)

ARBs, such as ***candesartan***, ***losartan***, and ***valsartan***; are often used as second line agents in patients who cannot tolerate ACE inhibitors. The mechanism of action for ARBs is through the blocking of angiotensin II receptors found in the kidney, thereby preventing the synthesis of aldosterone and lowering blood pressure and cardiac workload.

## Beta-Blockers

Beta-blockers are beta receptor antagonists that decrease heart rate and workload. Examples include ***bisoprolol*** and ***metoprolol***. Beta-blockers competitively block beta-receptors found in the heart and adrenal glands, in turn decreasing sympathetic activity and lowering heart rate and contractility.

## Loop Diuretics

For patients with advanced heart failure, lower limb edema can be seen in almost all cases and therefore, diuretics are commonly used to address the water retention with the goal of decreasing cardiac workload.

A conventional group of diuretics often used are the loop diuretics, such as ***furosemide*** and ***bumetanide***. These diuretics act on the ascending limb of the loop of Henle in the renal medulla by inhibiting the sodium-potassium-chloride cotransporter, causing a decrease of interstitial osmolality in the medulla of the kidney and decreasing the ability for the collecting duct to reabsorb water. As a result, water is excreted out of the body.

## Aldosterone Antagonists

Aldosterone antagonists such as ***spironolactone*** and ***eplerenone***, target the renin-angiotensinogen-angiotensin-system (RAAS) by inhibiting aldosterone receptors in the distal convoluted tubules and collecting ducts resulting in a decrease in blood pressure and cardiac workload.

## Vasodilators

Vasodilators, such as ***hydralazine***, act by relaxing smooth muscles surrounding arteries and causing vasodilation. The vasodilation leads to a decrease in vessel wall resistance, which then lowers blood pressure and afterload.

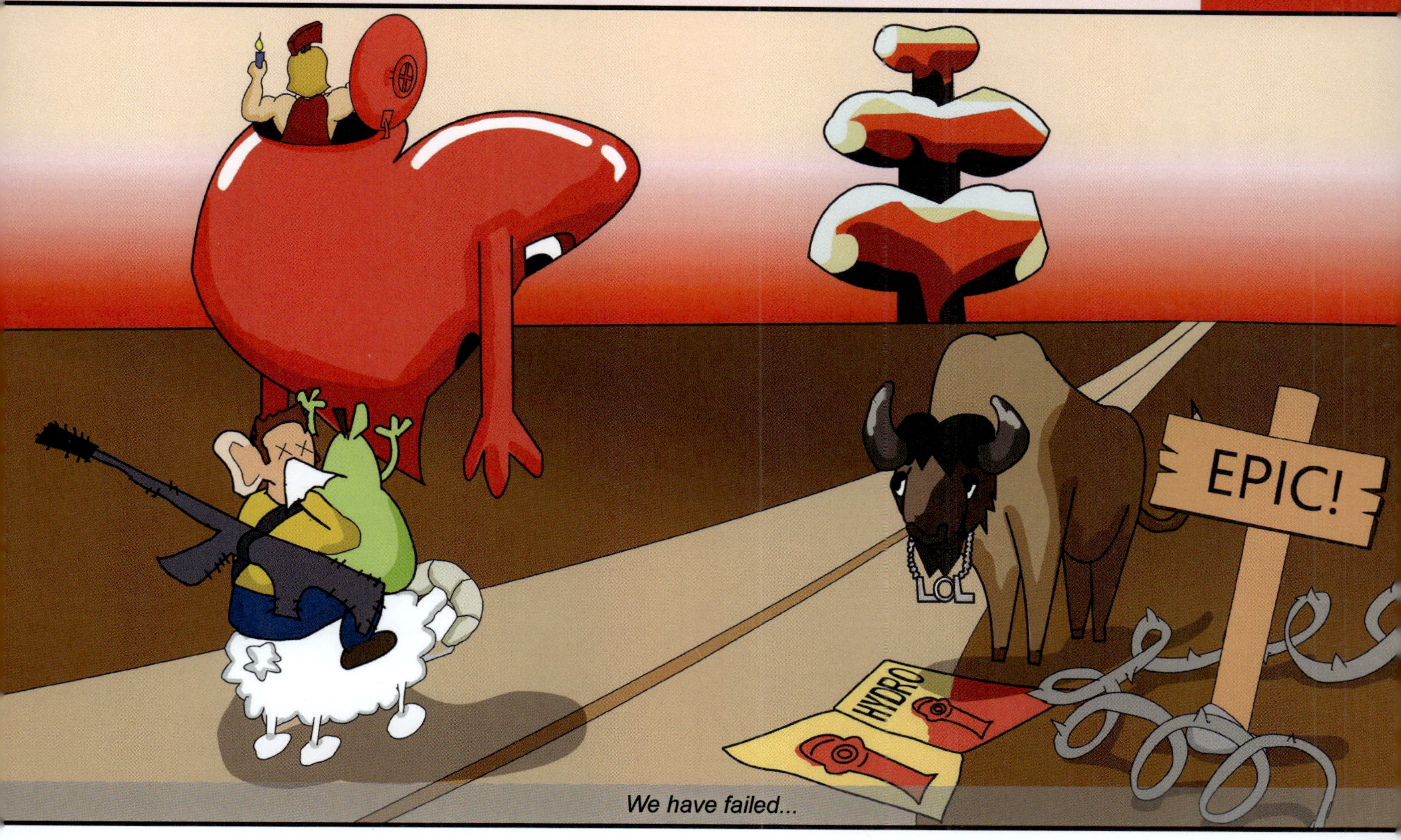


## HEART FAILURE

*The depressed heart reminds you that this picture is about heart failure!*

### ACE Inhibitors

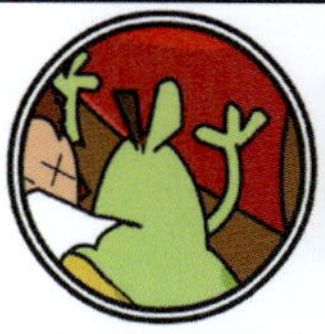
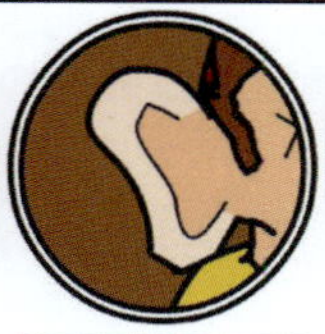
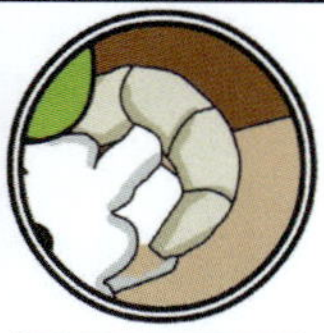

*"Pear-ill"* **Perindopril**

*"Listen-ill"* **Lisinopril**

*"Ram-ill"* **Ramipril**

### Angiotensin Receptor Blockers

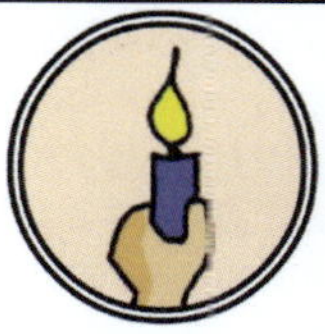
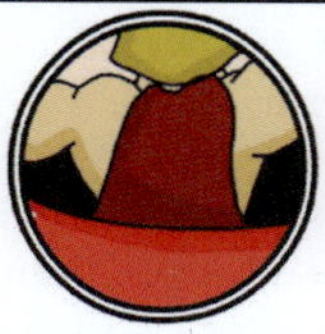
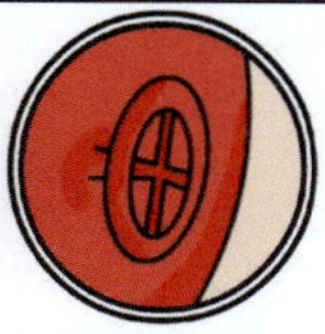

*"Candle-Spartan"* **Candesartan**

*"Low-Spartan"* **Losartan**

*"Valve-Spartan"* **Valsartan**

### Beta Blockers

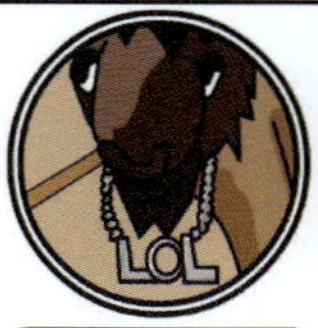

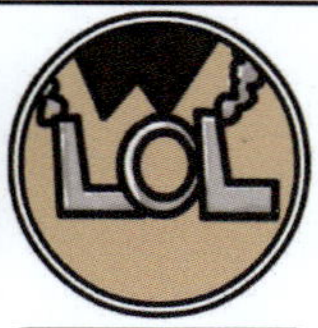


*"Bison-LOL"* **Bisoprolol**

*"Metal-LOL"* **Metoprolol**

### Loop Diuretics

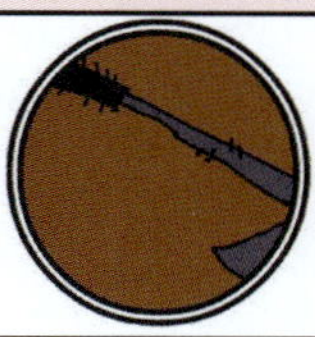
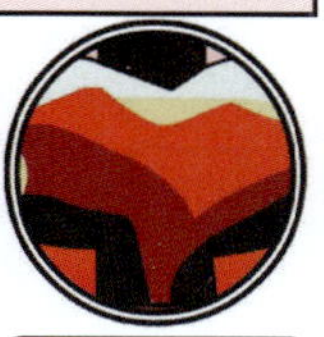

*"Fur-Semi [automatic]"* **Furosemide**

*"Boom"* **Bumetanide**

### Aldosterone Antagonists

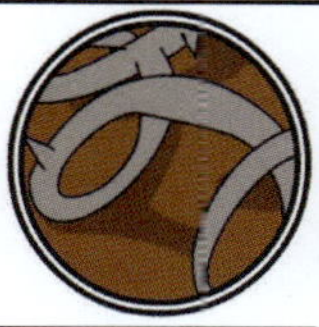
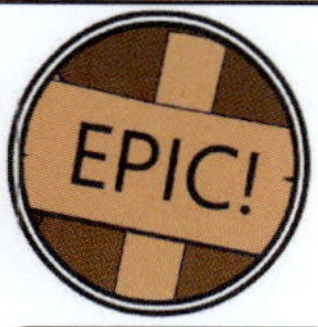


*"Spira."* **Spironolactone**

*"EPIC"* **Eplerenone**

### Vasodilators

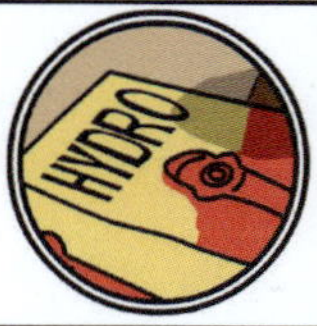


*"Hydro-Magazine"* **Hydralazine**

# DIURETICS

**Indications for diuretics:** CCF, nephrotic syndrome, renal disease, hypertension.

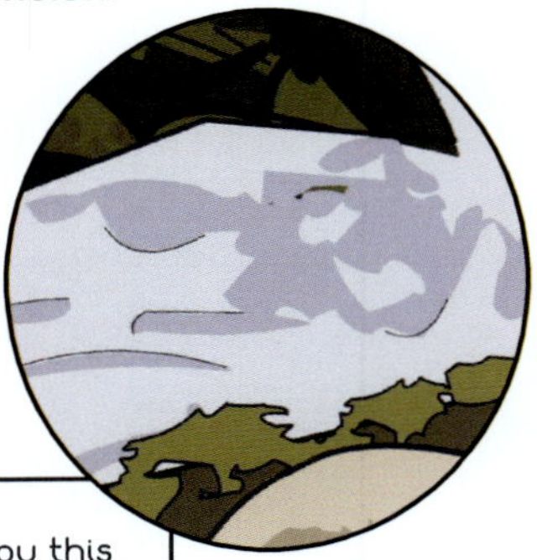

The flowing stream reminds you this picture is about diuretics!

**DIURETICS** are a class of drugs that facilitate water excretion from the body through urine. Although each drug varies in their mechanism of action, the target organ of diuretics are the kidneys. Diuretics are mainly used in patients who suffer from overload of fluid in the body due to various medical conditions, such as congestive heart failure.

## Loop Diuretics

***Furosemide*** and ***bumetanide*** are example of loop diuretics. Loop diuretics work by binding to the sodium-potassium-chloride cotransporter in the ascending loop of Henle in the kidney. This causes a decrease in interstitial osmolality in the renal medulla, and leads to more water excreted out of the body in urine.

Loop diuretics are indicated in diseases associated with fluid overload such as cardiac insufficiency, brain or lung edema, liver cirrhosis, and hypertension. The use of loop diuretics should be monitored in patients with electrolyte imbalance or cardiac arrhythmia because it has been linked to hyponatremia and hypokalemia. Besides that, loop diuretics are also known to be able to cause ototoxicity, tinnitus, and rarely, deafness.

## Thiazide Diuretics

***Hydrochlorothiazide***, ***bendroflumethiazide*** and ***metolazone*** are examples of thiazide diuretics. Thiazide diuretics act on the distal convoluted tubule (DCT) of the kidney nephron, where they inhibit the sodium-chloride symporter on the luminal membrane. As a result, sodium is unable to be resorbed. Because water follows sodium, water stays in the lumen with sodium, and is excreted in urine. Thiazides are often used in the treatment of uncomplicated hypertension and edema.

## Carbonic Anhydrase Inhibitors

***Acetazolamide*** and ***methazolamide*** are examples of carbonic anhydrase inhibitors. Carbonic anhydrase inhibitors are a class of diuretics that inhibit the enzyme carbonic anhydrase and act on the proximal tubule of the nephron. These medications inhibit the formation of water and carbon dioxide from carbonic acid, ultimately leading to water and sodium bicarbonate excretion in the urine.

Although carbonic anhydrase inhibitors possess diuretic properties, their effect is only minimal when compared to other diuretics. Clinical uses include treatment of glaucoma (topical), epilepsy, and altitude sickness.

## Potassium Sparing Diuretics

There are two groups of potassium sparing diuretics: aldosterone antagonists, such as ***spironolactone*** and ***eplerenone***, and sodium channel blockers, like ***amiloride***. Unlike loop and thiazide diuretics, these medications do not cause a loss of potassium.

Aldosterone antagonists exert their effect by inhibiting resorption of sodium into the collecting duct of the kidney. Furthermore, by competitively binding to basolateral aldosterone receptors, it blocks sodium transportation into the interstitium and potassium out into the cells.

Sodium channel blockers inhibit luminal sodium channels in the collecting tubule and collecting duct of the nephron. Usually, sodium from these channels would be used with the sodium potassium ATPase on the basolateral membrane, leading to potassium being transported out of the interstitium.

With both groups, the end result is a retention of potassium and an increase in sodium and water excretion. With this in mind, one of the main side effects of potassium sparing diuretics is hyperkalemia. Patients with electrolyte imbalances, such as those post-cardiac arrest, may be at increased risk of hyperkalemia with the use of these diuretics.

## Osmotic Diuretics

***Mannitol*** is an osmotic diuretic that is used for the regulation of blood volume in the body. Its clinical uses include glaucoma and emergency treatment of intracranial hypertension.

Mannitol is a sugar that is not reabsorbed by the kidney, therefore, it increases the renal osmolality of luminal fluid as it passes through the collecting duct system. This results in the pulling of water through osmotic pressure differences in the nephron and excretion of water out of the body.

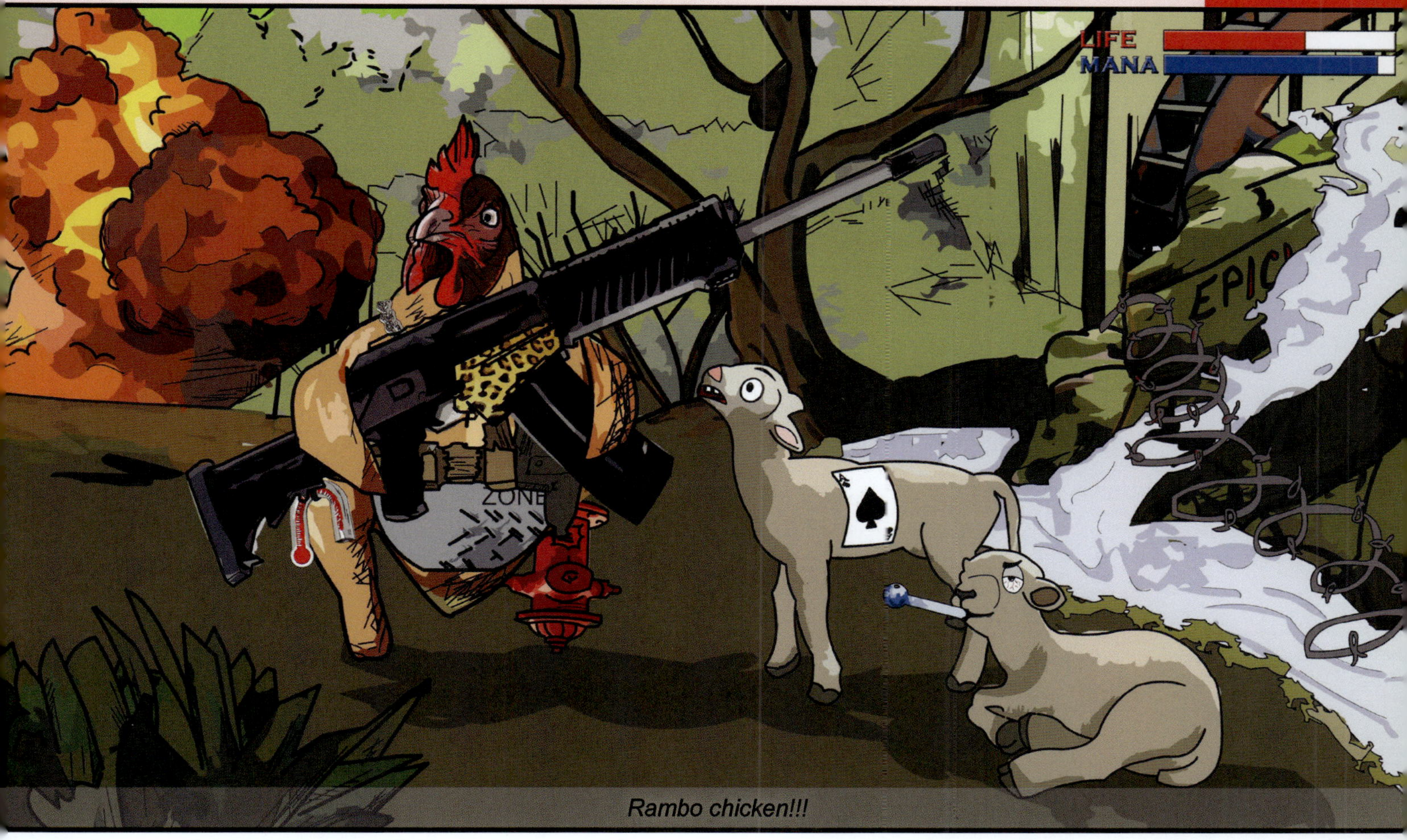

Rambo chicken!!!

# DIURETICS

*The flowing stream reminds you this picture is about diuretics!*

## Loop Diuretics

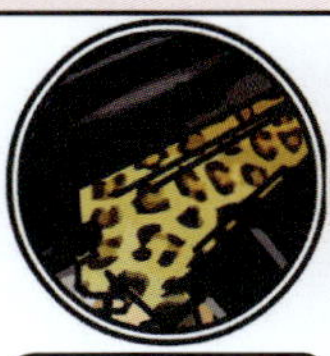
"Fur-Semi"
**Furosemide**

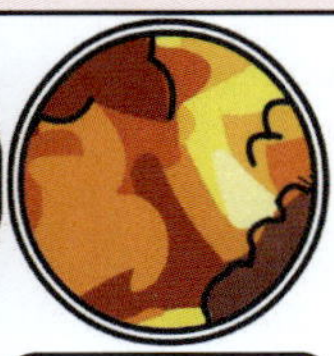
"Boom"
**Bumetanide**

## Thiazide Diuretics

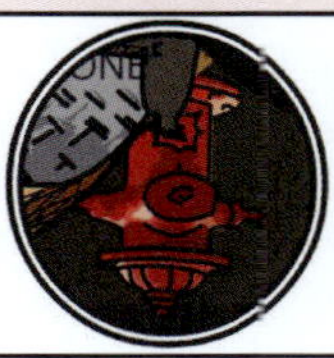

"Hydro-Thigh"
**Hydrochlorothiazide**

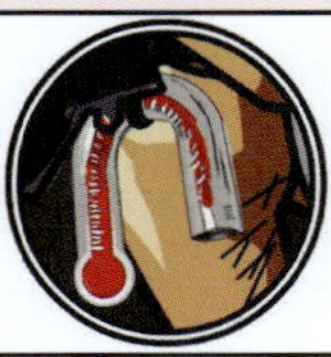
"Bend-Flu-Thigh"
**Bendroflumethiazide**

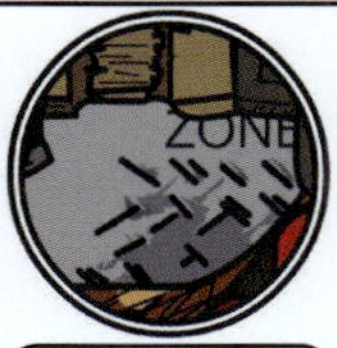

"Metal-Zone"
**Metolazone**

## Carbonic Anhydrase Inhibitors

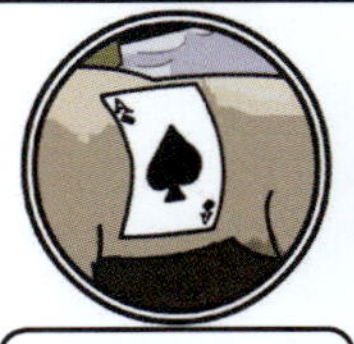
"Ace-Lamb"
**Acetazolamide**

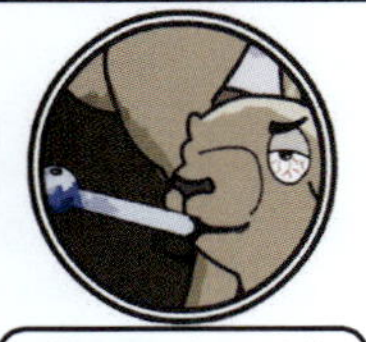
"Meth-Lamb"
**Methazolamide**

## Potassium Sparing Diuretics

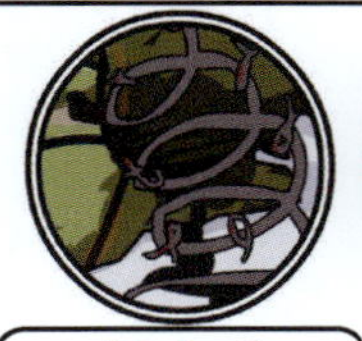
"Spiral"
**Spironolactone**

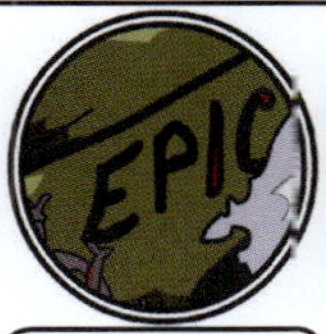

"EPIC"
**Eplerenone**

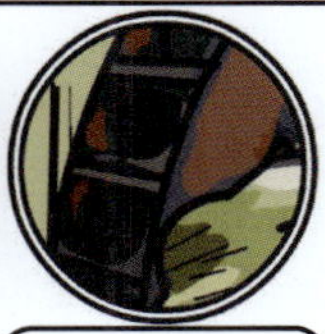
"A-Mill"
**Amiloride**

aldosterone antagonist

## Osmotic Diuretics

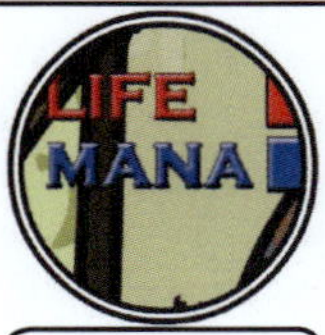

"MANA"
**Mannitol**

# ANGINA

**Indications for anginal medications:** angina (chest pain, tightness, pressure, squeezing).

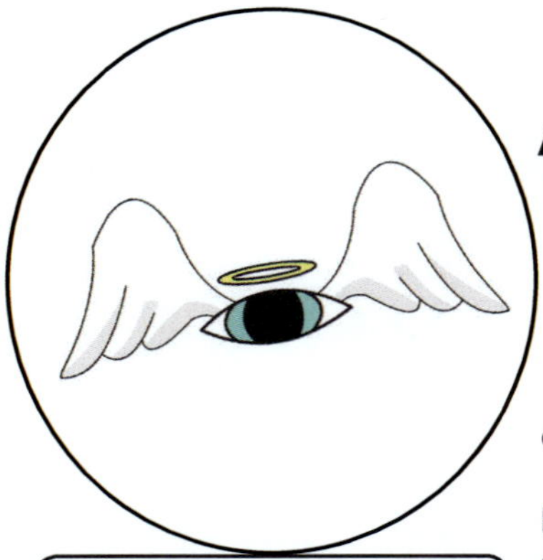

The angel-eye reminds you this picture is about angina.

**ANGINA PECTORIS** is the most common clinical presentation seen in patients who suffer from cardiovascular disease. It is classically defined as retrosternal pain brought on by poor blood flow to the heart, typically caused by ischemia of the myocardial tissues. This pain often radiates from the chest to the shoulder, neck region, or to one or both arms.

Modifying risk factors, such as stopping smoking, encouraging weight loss, exercise, and controlling hypertension and diabetes are important in treatment.

Pharmacological treatment is used in angina to relieve chest pain and prevent complications from occurring, these include nitrates, beta-blockers, calcium channel blockers, and antiplatelet agents.

## Nitrates

For symptomatic relief of angina pectoris, nitrates are often used - common examples include ***glyceryl trinitrate (GTN)*** and ***isosorbide dinitrate (ISDN)***.

The main goal of nitrates are to decrease oxygen demand of the heart muscles. Nitrates cause dilation of veins and decreases the volume of blood flowing back into the heart, which leads to less exertion on the heart muscles. Nitrates can be classified into short-acting and long-acting. The former is taken sublingually to relieve acute chest pain, while the latter is taken for prevention of angina.

## Beta-Blockers

***Atenolol*** and ***metoprolol*** are beta-1 receptor selective beta-blockers that act primarily on the heart, leading to a decrease in heart rate and cardiac output, and ultimately lowering oxygen demand of the myocardial tissues.

Side effects include hypotension, bradycardia, insomnia, dizziness, and/or abdominal discomfort.

## Calcium Channel Blockers

Calcium channel blockers decrease oxygen demand on the heart by decreasing the frequency of electrical impulses of the heart nodes, decreasing the strength of contraction of the heart, and also by dilating the smooth muscles of blood vessels. Some examples of calcium channel blockers are ***nifedipine***, ***amlodipine***, ***diltiazem***, and ***verapamil***.

Like other vasodilators, calcium channel blockers carry the risk of hypotension and should be avoided in patients who have low blood pressure.

## Antiplatelets

In order to prevent thrombus reformation, antiplatelet agents such as ***aspirin*** or ***clopidogrel*** are often used. Aspirin irreversibly inhibits cyclooxygenase enzymes, preventing the formation of prostaglandins and thromboxanes which are needed for platelet aggregation. Clopidogrel acts by inhibiting the adenosine diphosphate (ADP) receptor on platelet cell membranes leading to inhibition of platelet aggregation.

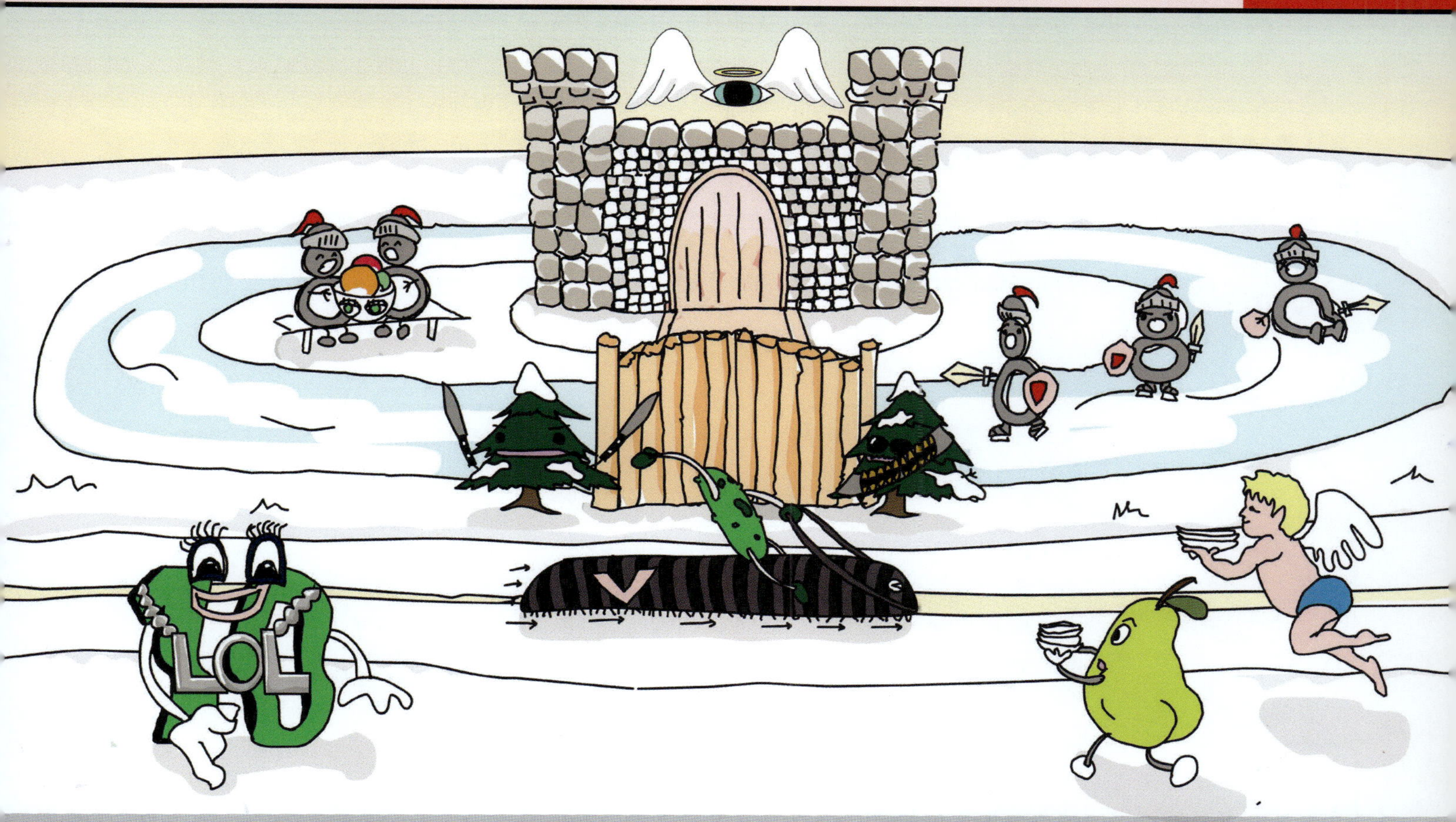

*Welcome to angina castle!*

## ANGINA

☞ *The angel-eye reminds you this picture is about angina.*

### Nitrates

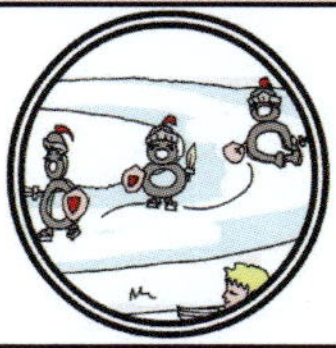

*"Glide-Tri-Knight-Eight"*
**Glyceryl trinitrate (GTN)**

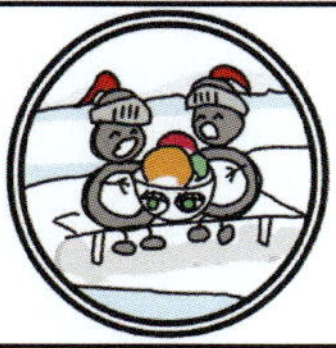

*"Sorbet-Di-Knight-Eight"*
**Isosobide Dinitrate (ISDN)**

### Beta Blockers

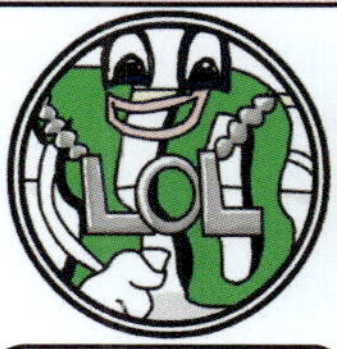

*"A-Ten-LOL"*
**Atenolol**

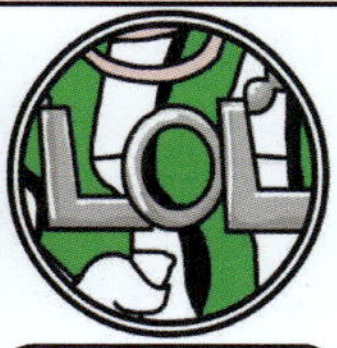

*"Metal-LOL"*
**Metoprolol**

### Calcium Channel Blockers

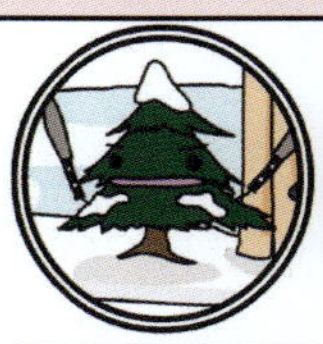

*"Knife-Pine"*
**Nifedipine**

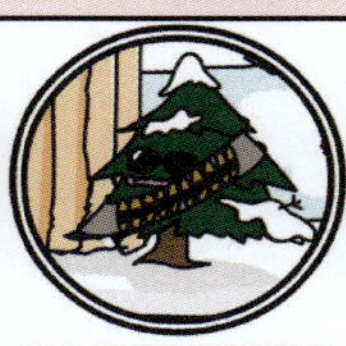

*"Ammo-Pine"*
**Amlodipine**

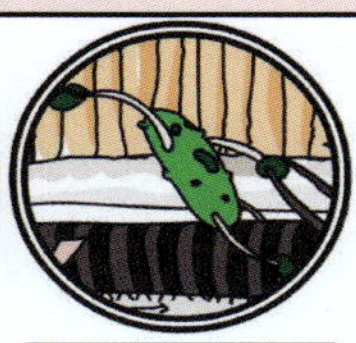

*"Dill"*
**Diltiazem**

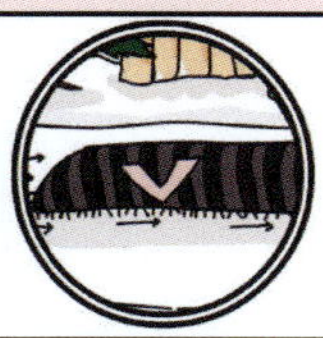

*"Very-[fast] Millipede"*
**Verapamil**

dihydropyridines

Benzothiazepines.

phenylalkilamine

### Antiplatelets

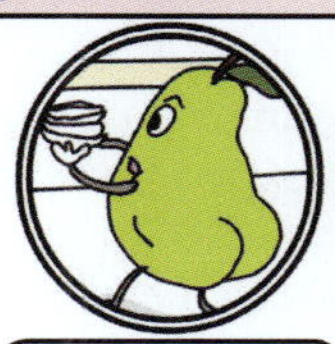

*"Ass-Pear"*
**Aspirin**

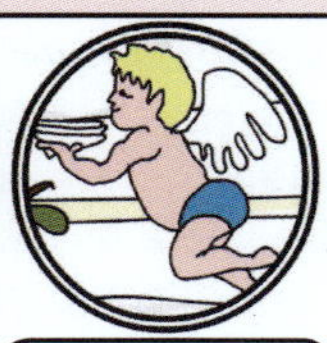

*"Cupid"*
**Clopidogrel**

ADPR

# LIPID LOWERING DRUGS

**Indications for lipid lowering drugs:** hyperlipidemia, hypercholesterolemia, coronary artery disease.

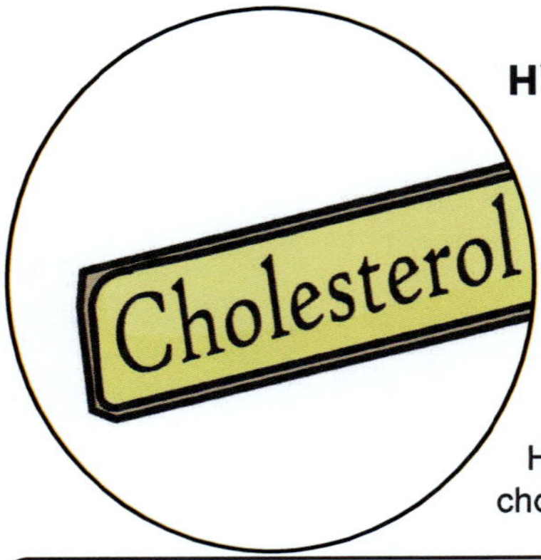


**HYPERLIPIDEMIA** is defined as abnormally elevated levels of cholesterol in the blood.

As cholesterol molecules are insoluble in the blood, they are carried around in the body by transporters known as lipoproteins. As such, lipoprotein levels are used as a measurable parameter of cholesterol levels in the blood.

Conventionally, high density lipoproteins (HDL) and low density lipoproteins (LDL) are used as markers. The LDLs transport fat cells from the liver and deposits them on the arterial wall, while HDLs do the opposite. The main goal of treatment is to raise HDL levels and/or lower LDL levels in the blood, and this is done using statins, fibrates, cholesterol absorbing inhibitors, ion exchange resins, and b-vitamins.

The cholesterol mines remind you this picture is about lipid lowering drugs!

## Statins

The most common group of drugs used to treat hyperlipidemia are statins (also known as HMG-CoA reductase inhibitors), such as ***atorvastatin***, ***simvastatin*** and ***rosuvastatin***.

Statins inhibit the enzyme HMG-CoA reductase and stops the formation of mevalonate, a crucial molecule necessary for cholesterol formation. Statins can also increase the re-uptake of LDL via synthesis of LDL receptors in the liver. Statin use is associated with hepatotoxicity and rhabdomyolysis (especially if used together with fibrates or niacin).

## Fibrates

Fibrates, such as ***fenofibrate***, ***bezafibrate***, and ***gemfibrozil***; share a similar molecular structure to the anti-diabetic drug class thiazolidinediones, and therefore act via similar mechanisms.

Fibrates activate peroxisome proliferator-activated receptors (PPARs), specifically PPAR-α. PPARs are located in the cell nuclei, and when activated, they stimulate the transcription of genes responsible for lipid metabolism. Fibrates also act by upregulating lipoprotein lipase which leads to breakdown of triglycerides to free fatty acids, leading to lower levels of very low density lipoprotein (VLDL).

## Cholesterol Absorbing Inhibitors

Blood cholesterol levels can also be reduced by inhibiting the absorption of cholesterol in the intestine. ***Ezetimibe*** is a drug that acts through this mechanism. By preventing cholesterol absorption in the intestine, the liver compensates by absorbing more cholesterol and thereby reducing cholesterol levels in the systemic circulation. Drugs in this class are generally used as a second-line treatment in the case where statins and fibrates are ineffective or contraindicated.

## Ion Exchange Resins

Since fat absorption from the intestines requires bile, bile acid resins, like ***cholestyramine***, are used to prevent intestinal resorption of bile acids. These drugs form insoluble complexes with bile and cause them to be excreted in faecal matter. Patients who are at high risk of developing gallstones should avoid using these drugs due to a compensatory process from the gallbladder where bile acid secretion is increased.

## B-Vitamins

The last group of drugs used to treat hyperlipidemia are B-vitamins such as ***nicotinic acid***. Although the exact mechanism of action of nicotinic acid is not well understood, its clinical significance has long been proven. It is proposed that nicotinic acid acts by inhibiting lipolysis in adipose tissue. Side effects are a red, flushed face, hyperglycemia, and hyperuricemia.

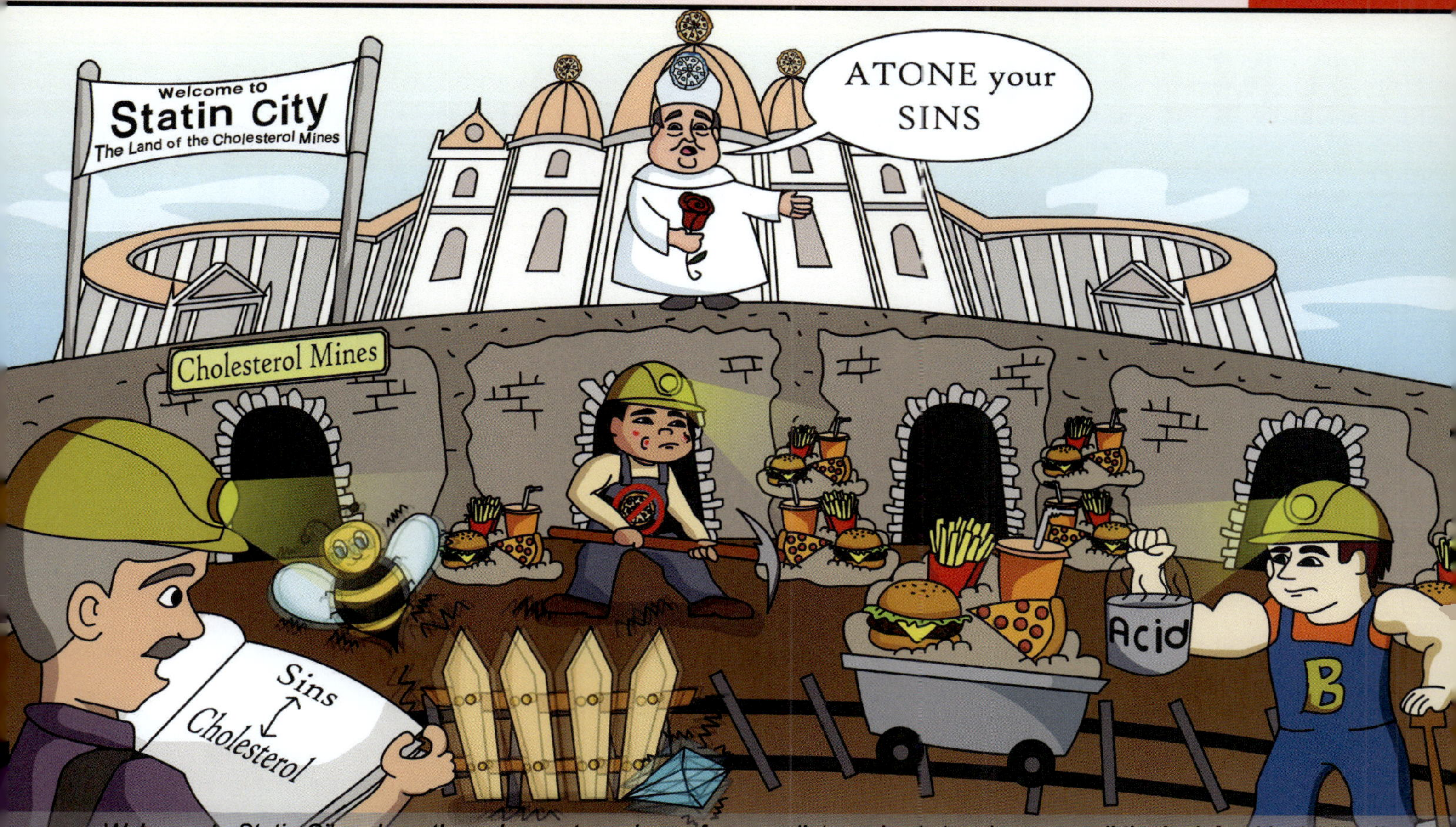


*Welcome to Statin City, where the only way to make up for your dietary sins is to mine away all the junk food in the land!*

## LIPID LOWERING DRUGS

☞ *The cholesterol mines remind you this picture is about lipid lowering drugs!*

### Statins

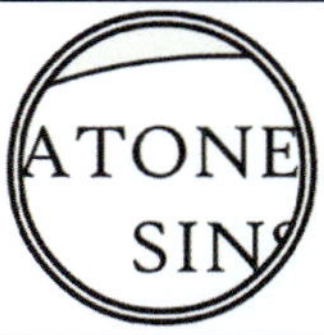


*"Atone-Statin [City]"*
**Atorvastatin**

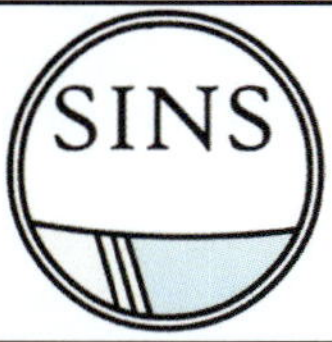


*"Sin-Statin [City]"*
**Simvastatin**

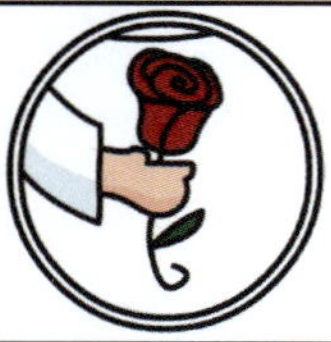

*"Rose-Statin [City]"*
**Rosuvastatin**

### Fibrates

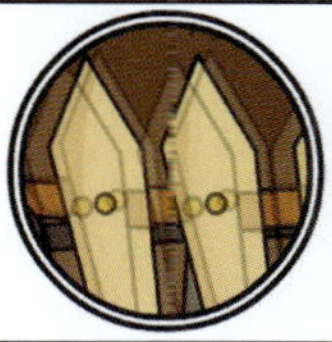

*"Fence-Vibrate"*
**Fenofibrate**

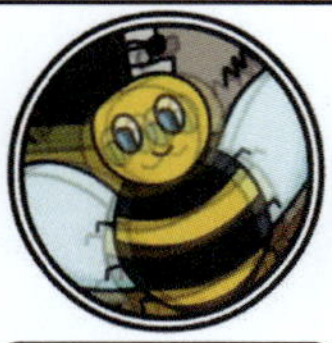

*"Bee-Vibrate"*
**Bezafibrate**

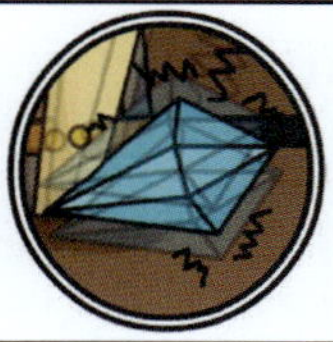

*"Gem-Vibrate"*
**Gemfibrozil**

### Cholesterol Absorption Inhibitors

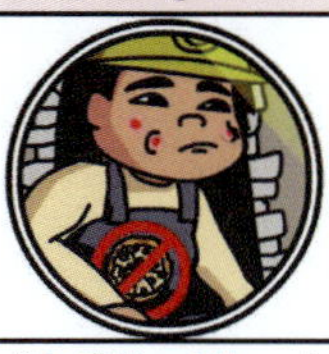

*"A-Zitty-Miner"*
**Ezetimibe**

### Ion Exchange Resins

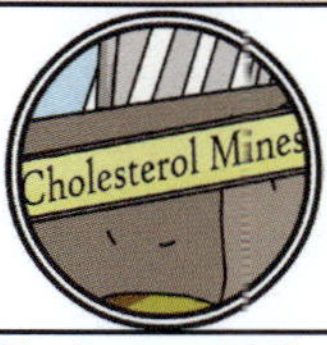


*"Cholesterol-Mine"*
**Cholestyramine**

### B Vitamins

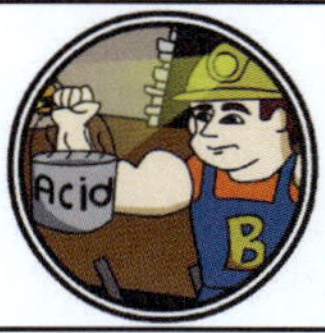


*"Tin-Acid"*
**Nicotinic Acid**

# ANTIDIABETIC MEDICATION

**Indications for antidiabetic medications:** diabetes type I and II.

**DIABETES MELLITUS** is a chronic disease characterized by elevated blood glucose levels and impaired ability to produce or react to the hormone insulin. Diabetic patients usually present with a variety of symptoms including frequent urination, excessive thirst, and increased appetite.

Generally, the disease is divided into two main categories known as type I and type II diabetes mellitus (DM). Type I DM is an autoimmune disease that causes a decrease in insulin production from the pancreas. Type II DM is thought to be caused by a combination of environmental and genetic factors, and is associated with insulin receptor insensitivity.

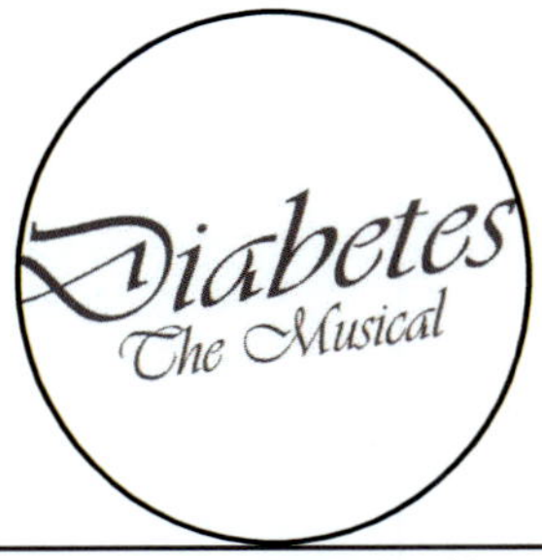


The picture "Diabetes the Musical" reminds you this picture is about antidiabetic medications.

## Insulin

Subcutaneous ***insulin*** injection is mainly indicated for Type I DM patients. This group of medication is categorized based on their onset and duration of action. Usually a short and intermediate acting insulin is combined and injected twice daily before meal time, or a long acting insulin may be administered in the morning followed by the short acting analogue during meal times. These analogues act by promoting glucose absorption at the peripheral tissues thereby keeping blood sugar levels closer to normal ranges. ***Lispro*** is an example of fast acting insulin, insulin suspended in ***zinc*** an intermediate acting, and ***glargine*** is an example of a long acting insulin.

## Biguanides

***Metformin*** is a ***biguanide*** commonly used as the first line treatment due to its ability to reduce cardiovascular morbidity and mortality. It acts by inhibiting gluconeogenesis in the liver and also increase glucose absorption in the peripheral tissues. Metformin activates AMP-activated protein kinase, which is needed for the inhibition of gluconeogenesis in liver.

## Sulfonylureas

***Sulfonylureas*** are a common group of drugs used for the treatment of Type II DM. Examples of sulfonylureas include ***gliclazide*** and ***glyburide*** (glibenclamide). These drugs are taken orally and act by closing ATP-sensitive K+ channels on beta-islet cells of the pancreas, eventually leading to release of insulin.

## Thiazolidinediones

***Thiazolidinediones*** help increase the sensitivity of insulin receptors at the peripheral cells. This is accomplished by stimulation of nuclear peroxisome proliferator-activated receptors (PPAR) gamma, which is responsible for the transcription of genes involved in carbohydrate metabolism among other functions. This group of drug is reserved for patients who fail to control their blood sugar levels by metformin and sulfonylureas. Examples: ***rosiglitazone*** and ***pioglitazone***

## Alpha Glucosidase Inhibitors

***Acarbose*** is an alpha-glucosidase inhibitor. Alpha-glucosidase is an enzyme needed to breakdown carbohydrates into simple chains. As a result, carbohydrates digestion will be stretched over a longer time frame to prevent a sudden peak of blood glucose level.

## Dipeptidyl Petidase-4 (DPP4) Inhibitors

***DPP4-Inhibitors*** act by inhibiting DDP-4, an enzyme responsible for the inactivation of incretins like GLP-1 and GIP. As a result, insulin will be synthesized and released whereas glucagon synthesis will be suppressed. The net effect is the lowering of blood sugar levels. Examples: ***saxagliptin*** and ***sitagliptin***.

## Sodium/Glucose Cotransporter 2 (SGLT-2) Inhibitors

***SGLT-2 inhibitors*** differ by preventing glucose reabsorption in the kidney, thereby leading to a net loss of glucose in the urine. This group of drugs has been proven to decrease body weight and control blood pressure. Example: ***canagliflozin***.

## Glucagon-Like Peptide-1 (GLP-1) Agonists

***GLP-1 agonists*** can help normalize blood sugar levels by triggering the release of insulin in the beta-islet cells of the pancreas. Example: ***exenatide***.

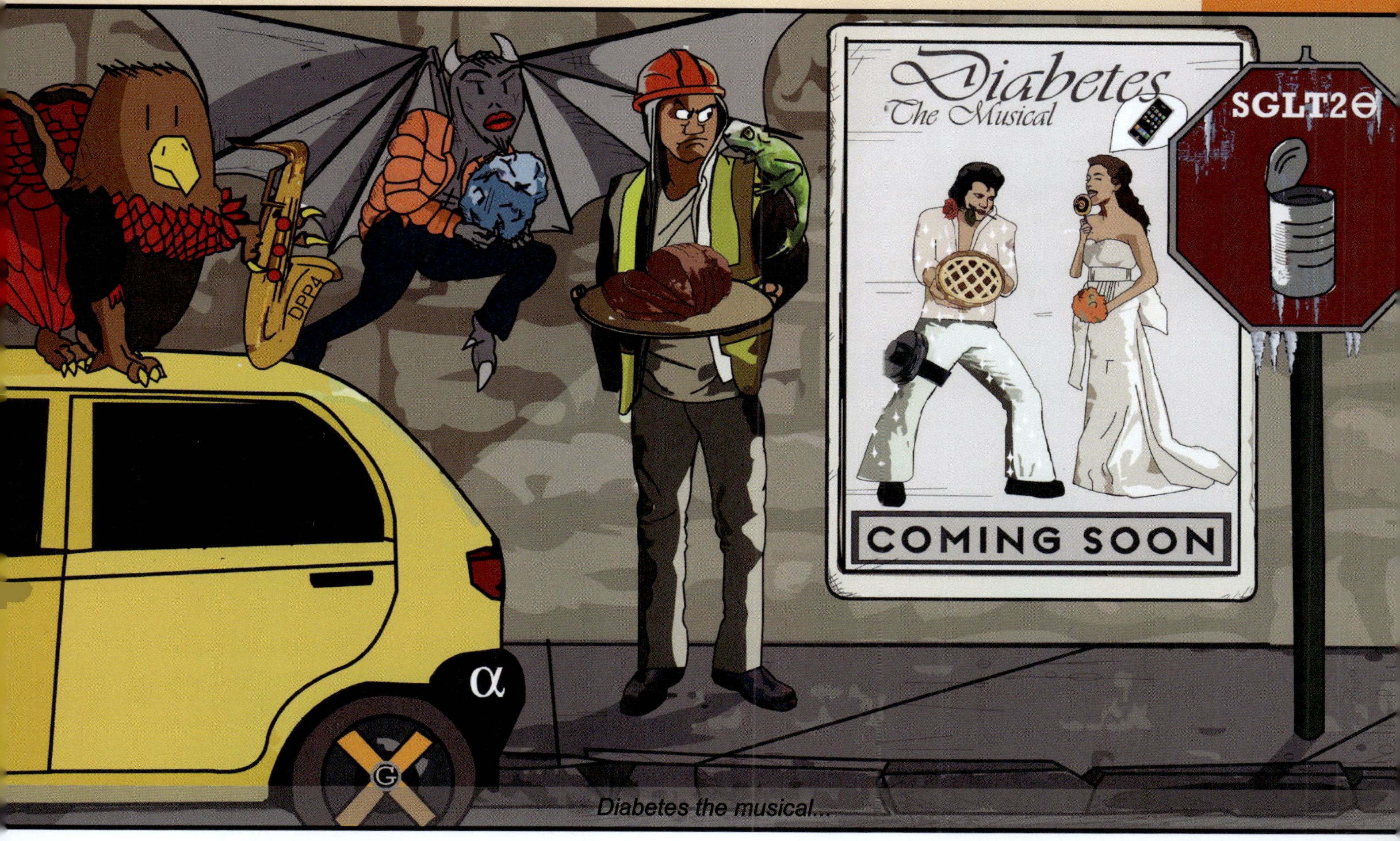


## ANTIDIABETIC MEDICATION

*The picture "Diabetes the Musical" reminds you this picture is about antidiabetic medications.*

### Insulins

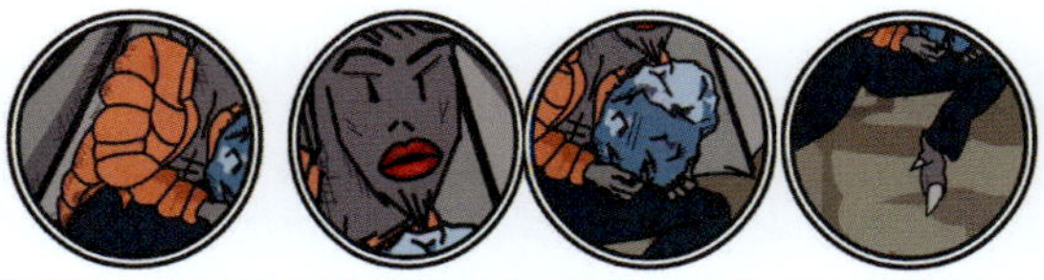

| | | | |
|---|---|---|---|
| *"Insulated [jacket]"* | *"Lips"* | *"Zinc"* | *"Gargoyle-Jean"* |
| **Insulin** | **Lispro** | **Zinc** | **Glargine** |

### Biguanides

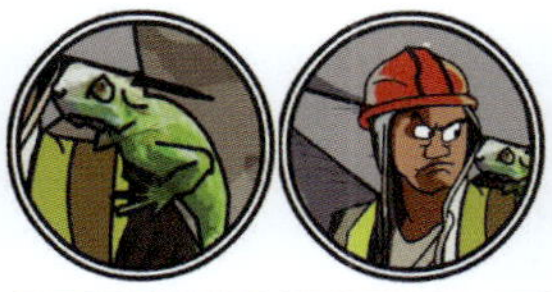

| | |
|---|---|
| *"Iguana"* | *"Meat-Foreman"* |
| **Biguanides** | **Metformin** |

### SGLT-2 Inhib.

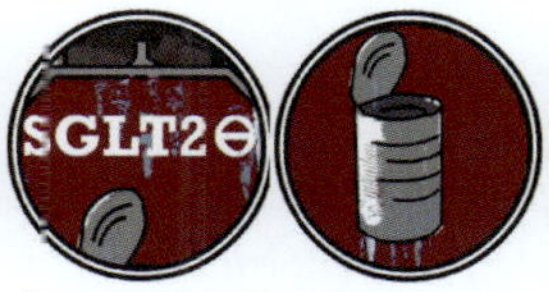

| | |
|---|---|
| *"STOP"* | *"Can-Frozen"* |
| **SGLT-2** | **Canagliflozin** |

### GLP-1 Agonists

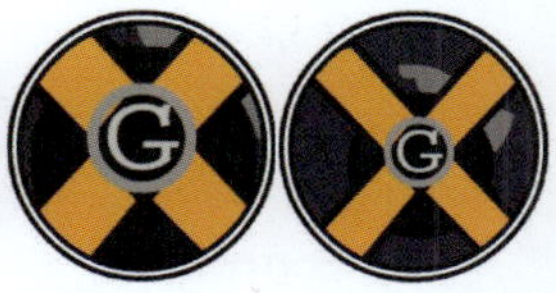

| | |
|---|---|
| *"G"* | *"X"* |
| **GLP-1 agonists** | **Exenatide** |

### Sulfonylureas

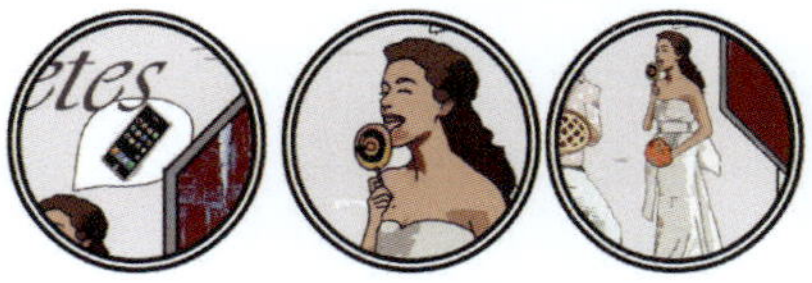

| | | |
|---|---|---|
| *"Cell-Phone"* | *"Lick"* | *"Bride"* |
| **Sulfonylureas** | **Gliclazide** | **Glyburide** |

### Thiazolidinediones

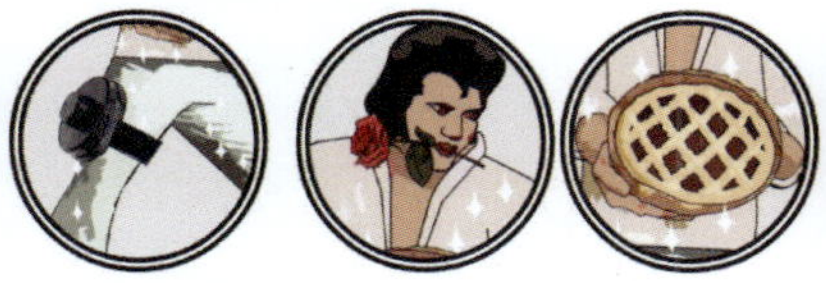

| | | |
|---|---|---|
| *"Thigh-Lid"* | *"Rose-Glitter"* | *"Pie-Glitter"* |
| **Thiazolidinediones** | **Rosiglitazone** | **Pioglitazone** |

### DPP-4 Inhibitors

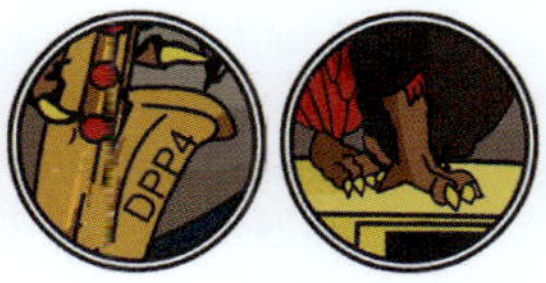

| | |
|---|---|
| *"Sax-Gryffin"* | *"Sitting-Gryffin"* |
| **Saxagliptin** | **Sitagliptin** |

### α-Glucosidase I.

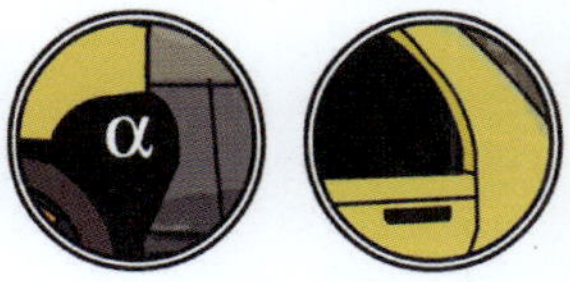

| | |
|---|---|
| *"Alpha"* | *"A Car"* |
| **Alpha Glucosidase Inhibitors** | **Acarbose** |

# STEROIDS

**Indications for steroids:** antiinflammatory uses, anaphylaxis, septic shock, cerebral oedema, analgesia adjunct, asthma, COPD, adrenal insufficiency.

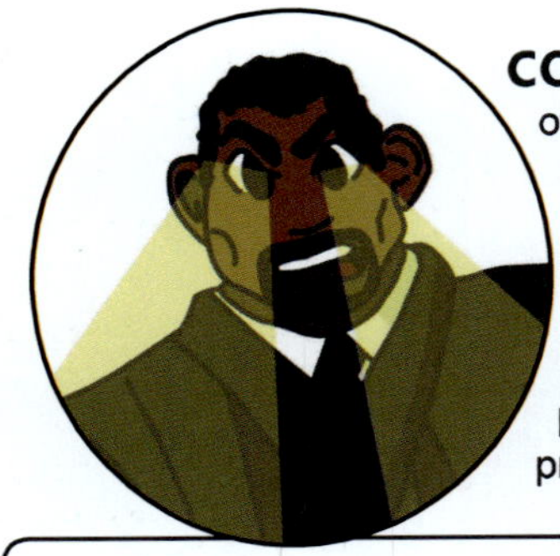

The stare of the judge reminds you this picture is about steroids!

**CORTICOSTEROIDS** are a class of steroid hormones that are responsible for the regulation of a wide range of physiological processes. They are produced both naturally in the body, and synthetically to be used as medications. Natural corticosteroids can be classified into glucocorticoids and mineralocorticoids. Physiologically, these compounds are synthesized in the adrenal glands and released into the bloodstream in response to physical or emotional stress.

Corticosteroids act by binding to the glucocorticoid receptor, which in turn upregulates the production of anti-inflammatory proteins and down-regulates the production of proinflammatory proteins.

Side effects of steroid use are well documented and include cushingoid appearance, acne, increased appetite, weight gain, hirsutism, hypertension, adrenal cortex suppression, sleep-disturbances, cataracts, osteoporosis, diabetes, and growth retardation.

## Glucocorticoid

A naturally occurring glucocorticoid is ***cortisol***. It is a natural stress hormone characterized by its ability to facilitate protein catabolism, gluconeogenesis, growth, and anti-inflammatory effects.

## Mineralocorticoid

***Aldosterone*** is a mineralocorticoid produced in the body that is mainly involved with sodium and water reabsorption in the distal convoluted tubules of the kidney. It is a key component in the renin-angiotensin-aldosterone system (RAAS) that is responsible for regulating the body's blood pressure.

## Synthetic Corticosteroids

When used as a medication, cortisol is known as ***hydrocortisone***. It comes in the form of an oral tablet, topical cream or injectable solution. It is used in many ailments including asthma, COPD, adrenocortical insufficiency, rheumatoid arthritis, dermatitis, and in the management of severe hypersensitivity reactions such as anaphylaxis.

***Betamethasone*** is a corticosteroid that can be administered orally, topically, intravenously, or through inhalation. It is used mainly for the treatment of rheumatic diseases such as rheumatoid arthritis or systemic lupus erythematosus. Betamethasone is also used to manage allergic conditions like dermatitis, psoriasis and bronchial asthma.

***Fluticasone*** is primarily used as a inhaled corticosteroid for the prevention of asthma, but can also be used as a topical anti-inflammatory.

***Clobetasone*** is another corticosteroid widely used in dermatology and ophthalmology. It is effective for the treatment of skin diseases such as eczema, dermatitis, and psoriasis. It can also be used in the form of eye drops to treat Sjogren's syndrome, a type of autoimmune disease that causes dry eyes.

***Beclomethasone*** is primarily used as an inhaled agent for the long term treatment of asthma, however, it is also used as a topical cream for dermatitis and has an oral form that can be used to treat inflammatory bowel disease (IBD).

***Budesonide*** is primarily used as an inhaled corticosteroid used for the management of bronchial asthma and chronic obstructive pulmonary disease. It can also be used to treat allergic rhinitis, nasal polyps, and IBD. It suppresses the immune system by acting as an agonist at glucocorticoid receptors and preventing various inflammatory processes.

***Prednisolone*** is used for the treatment of wide spectrum of diseases associated with allergic reactions, inflammatory bowel disease, autoimmune diseases, and in some cases, cancer. It is usually taken orally but is also available as injectable suspensions or topical creams.

***Fludrocortisone*** has one of the strongest anti-inflammatory properties compared to other corticosteroids. It is a short-acting glucocorticoid with a similar half-life to hydrocortisone. It is used mainly for the treatment of conditions associated with adrenal insufficiency and congenital adrenal hyperplasia. It can also be used to diagnose Conn's syndrome through the fludrocortisone suppression test.

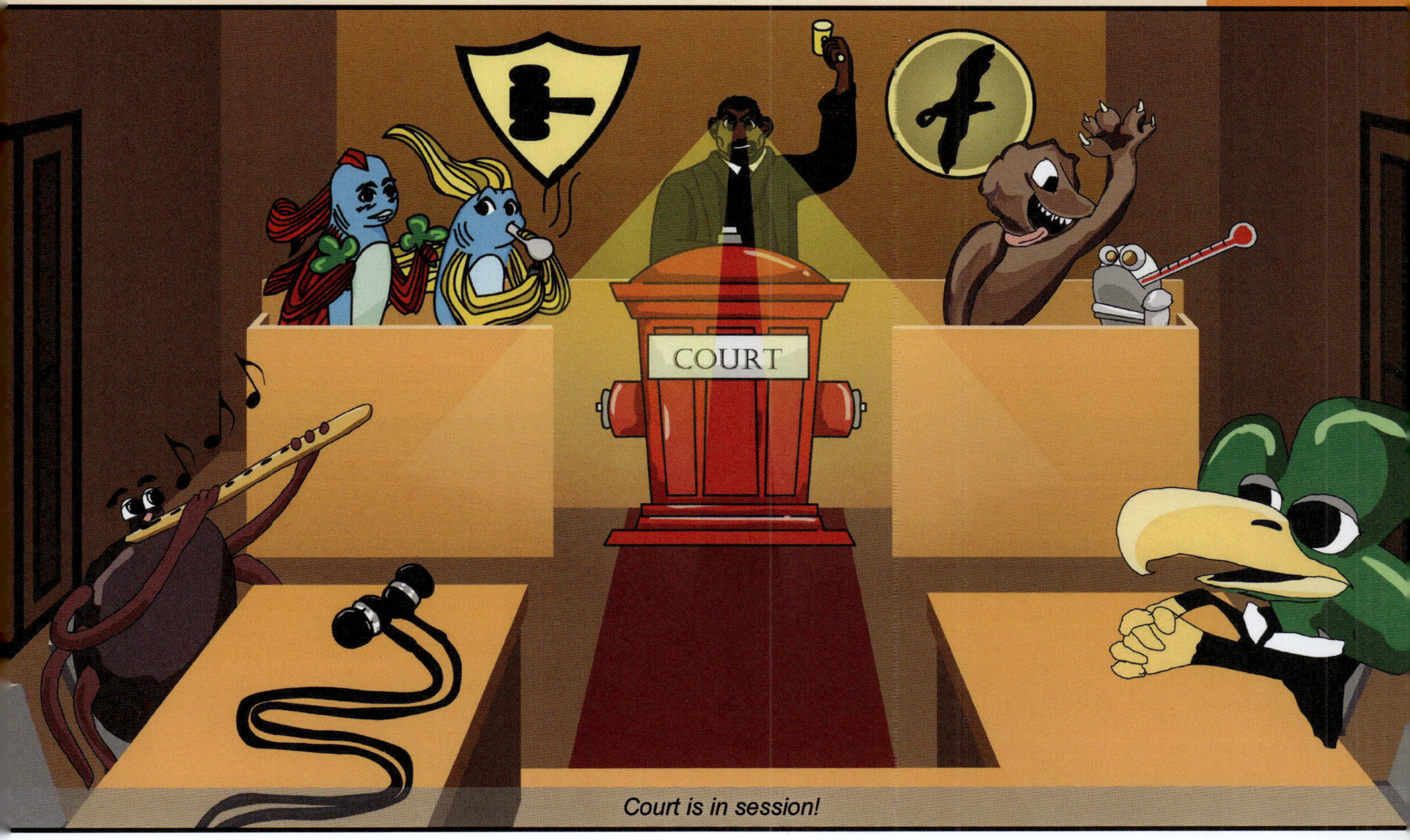


*Court is in session!*

## STEROIDS

*The stare of the judge reminds you this picture is about steroids!*

### Glucocorticoids

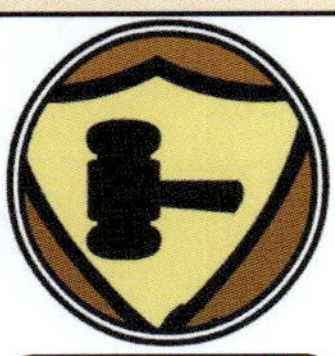

*"Court"*
**Cortisol**

### Mineralocorticoids

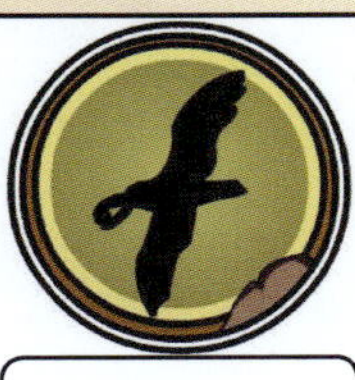

*"Albatross-Stone"*
**Aldosterone**

### Synthetic Corticosteroids

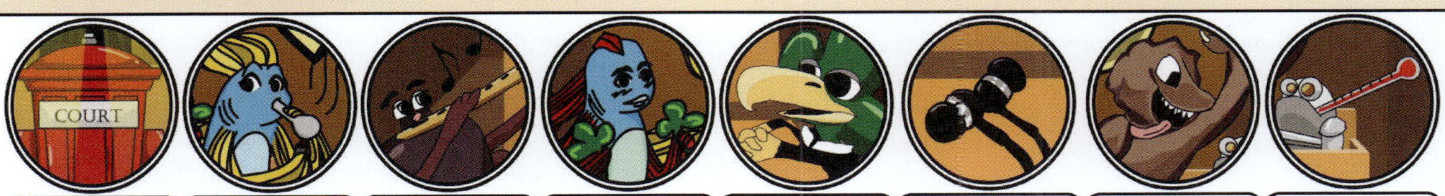


| | | | | | | | |
|---|---|---|---|---|---|---|---|
| *"Hydro-Court"* | *"Betta-Meth"* | *"Flute-Tick"* | *"Clover-Betta"* | *"Beak-Clover"* | *"[Ear]-Buds"* | *"Predator"* | *"Flu-Drone"* |
| **Hydrocortisone** | **Betamethasone** | **Fluticasone** | **Clobetasone** | **Beclomethasone** | **Budesonide** | **Prednisolone** | **Fludrocortisone** |

*Betta refers to a type of fish called the Betta-Fish.*

# PEPTIC ULCER DISEASE

**Indications for PUD medications:** PUD, gastritis.

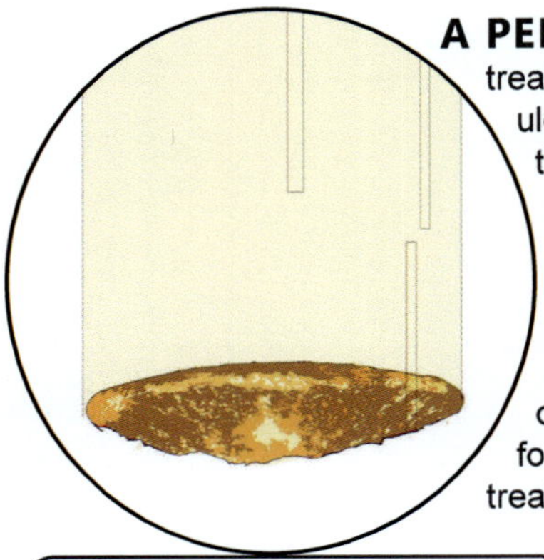

**A PEPTIC ULCER** is a break in the mucosal lining of the stomach or small intestine. Without treatment, gastric secretions such as pepsin and hydrochloric acid can further erode the ulcer and consequent inflammation of the surrounding tissues can occur. In severe cases, the erosion can penetrate into the lamina propria and submucosal layer leading to gastric bleeding. Most peptic ulcers occur either in the duodenum or in the stomach. They may also take place in the lower portion of esophagus due to regurgitation of gastric contents. If left untreated, peptic ulcers may develop into malignancy. Most cases of peptic ulcer disease are due to Helicobacter pylori infection. Other secondary factors that contribute to PUD development include NSAIDs, stress, smoking, and excessive alcohol consumption. The goal of treatment is to control gastric acid secretions and provide time for the ulcer to heal. In the case of H. pylori infection, the use of antibiotics is part of the treatment regime.

The sun's crater reminds you of ulcers, which in turn reminds you that this picture is about peptic ulcer disease!

## Proton Pump Inhibitors (PPIs)

One of the most important medications needed to suppress acid secretion are the proton pump inhibitors (PPIs). They work by irreversibly blocking hydrogen-potassium-ATPase pumps found on parietal cells in the stomach. As gastric acid secretion is being reduced, the pH level of the stomach becomes less acidic and minimizes gastric mucosal damage. Examples of PPIs are ***omeprazole***, ***lansoprazole***, and ***pantoprazole***. PPIs are generally well tolerated and do not cause any serious side effects. Some mild side effects include nausea, vomiting and abdominal discomfort.

## H2 Receptor Blockers

The next class of drugs effective for the treatment of PUD are histamine H2-receptor blockers, such as ***cimetidine*** and ***ranitidine***. These drugs decrease stomach acid production through reversibly inhibiting H2-receptors found in gastric parietal cells. As a result, stomach acidity decreases due to lower hydrogen ion concentration. H2-receptor blockers can lead to side effects such as headache and abdominal discomfort. For people who are allergic to H2-receptor blockers, they might experience hypersensitivity reaction such as urticaria.

## Antacids

This class of drugs that works by increasing/neutralizing the pH level of the stomach. Antacids are available over the counter in the form of capsules, tablets, powders, chewable tablets and suspension. They are relatively well tolerated compared to other gastric acid inhibitors. Examples of antacids are ***sodium bicarbonate*** (***$NaHCO_3$***) and ***calcium carbonate*** (***$CaCO_3$***). Magnesium may cause diarrhea while calcium and aluminium containing antacids may lead to constipation. Long term use of this class of drug may lead to kidney stone formation or osteoporosis.

## Mucosal Protectants

***Misoprostol*** is a prostaglandin analogue that acts on gastric parietal cells to inhibit the secretion of gastric acid. It is often used for the prevention of stomach ulcers caused by NSAIDs.

***Sucralfate*** reacts with hydrochloric acid and form a cross-linking acid buffer that lasts up to 8 hours in a single dose. It is often used for the treatment of duodenal ulcers.

## Triple Therapy for H. Pylori

As for Helicobacter pylori infections, the treatment regime known as "Triple therapy" is usually used. Triple therapy involves the use of a PPI, ***amoxicillin*** and ***clarithromycin***. Patients who are allergic to penicillin can replace amoxicillin with metronidazole.

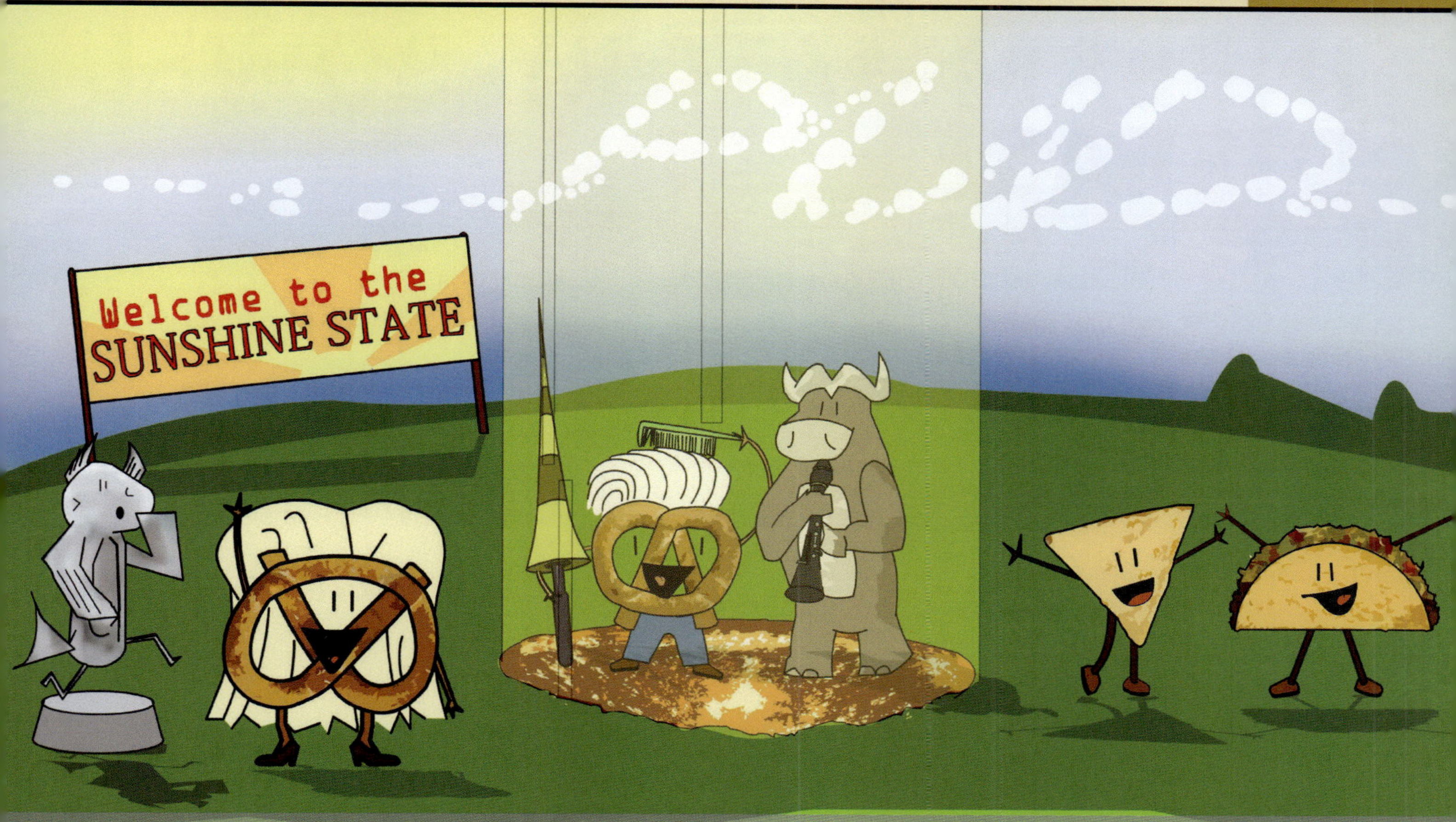


*Welcome to the sunshine state!*

## PEPTIC ULCER DISEASE

*The sun's crater reminds you of ulcers, which in turn reminds you that this picture is about peptic ulcer disease!*

### Proton Pump Inhibitors (PPI)

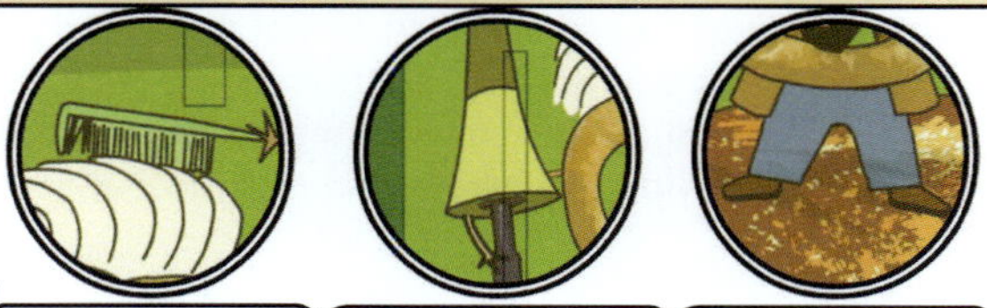

"Comb-Pretzel"
**Omeprazole**

"Lance-Pretzel"
**Lansoprazole**

"Pant-Pretzel"
**Pantoprazole**

### H2 Receptor Antagonists

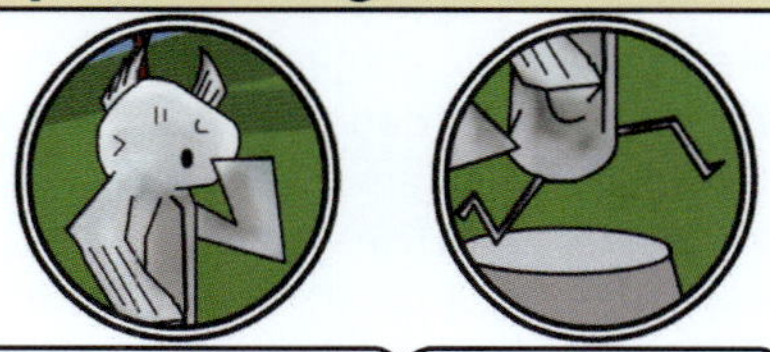

"Cement-Sardine"
**Cimetidine**

"Run-Sardine"
**Ranitidine**

### Antacids

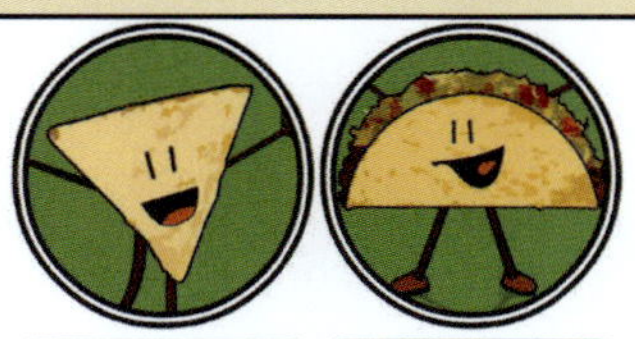

"NACHO"
**$NaHCO_3$**

"TACO"
**$CaCO_3$**

### Mucosal Protectants

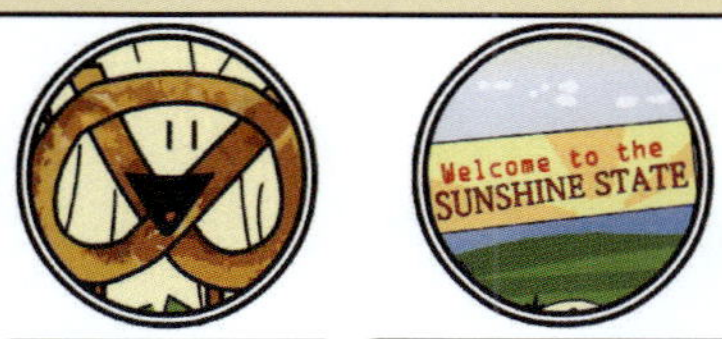


"Miss-Pretzel"
**Misoprostal**

"Sunshine-State"
**Sucralfate**

### Antibiotics

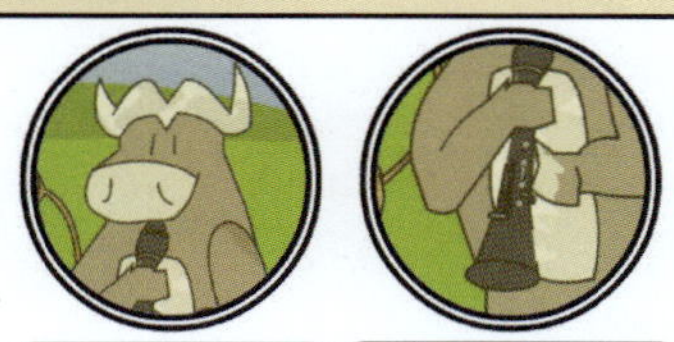

"An-Ox"
**Amoxicillin**

"Clarinet"
**Clarithromycin**

# INFLAMMATORY BOWEL DISEASE

**Indications for IBD medications:** Crohn's disease, ulcerative colitis.

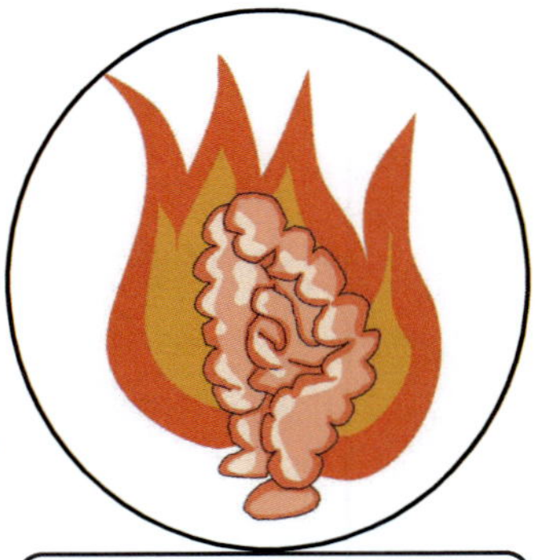

The bowel on fire reminds you this picture is about inflammatory bowel disease!

**INFLAMMATORY BOWEL DISEASE (IBD)** is a group of inflammatory conditions that involve the alimentary tract. It is comprised of Crohn's disease and ulcerative colitis, both of which have different clinical presentations and management approaches.

In Crohn's disease, inflammation may occur in any part of the gastrointestinal tract, from the mouth to the anus, and usually affects all layers of the bowel wall. Ulcerative colitis inflammation is usually confined to the colon and rectum, and only affects the inner lining of the colon.

The etiology of IBD is related to a combination of genetic and environmental factors, resulting in an autoimmune response in the gastrointestinal tract. Therefore, the aim of pharmacological intervention is to suppress the autoimmune response, to induce and maintain remission of inflammation, and to improve quality of life.

## Corticosteroids

Corticosteroids, such as ***prednisolone***, ***hydrocortisone*** and ***budesonide***; have anti-inflammatory and immune-suppressing effects, and are one of the most common classes of drugs used in the treatment of IBD.

Corticosteroids bind to glucocorticoid receptors forming a complex that interacts with DNA to inhibit transcription of inflammatory genes. As a result, production of inflammatory mediators such as platelet activating factor, leukotrienes, prostaglandins, histamine, and bradykinin will be reduced. Corticosteroids also decrease the production of cytokines such as interleukin-1, interleukin-2, interferon, and tumor necrosis factors (TNF). Long term use of corticosteroids is associated with the development of Cushing's syndrome and abrupt withdrawal can cause adrenal insufficiency.

## Aminosalicylates

Aminosalicylates, such as ***sulfasalazine*** and ***mesalazine*** (also known as 5-aminosalicylic acid or 5-ASA), act specifically in the bowel rather than targeting the whole body system, and lead to fewer systemic side effects compared to other drugs.

The exact mechanism of action of aminosalicylates is not fully understood, but may decrease inflammatory processes in the gut through the inhibition of cyclooxygenase, an enzyme responsible for the production of prostaglandins. Due to toxicity, aminosalicylates are contraindicated in children under two years of age and in patients with chronic kidney disease.

## Monoclonal Antibodies (mAb)

Monoclonal antibodies, such as ***infliximab*** and ***adalimumab***, act by binding to tumor necrosis factor (TNF)-alpha and prevent the activation of this pro-inflammatory molecule. Monoclonal antibodies can also induce the apoptosis of T-lymphocytes and monocytes, and downregulate other inflammatory molecules.

## Immunosuppressants

Immunosuppressants, such as ***azathioprine***, ***mercaptopurine***, and ***methotrexate***; can also be used to treat IBD.

***Azathioprine*** inhibits nucleic acid synthesis and suppresses cell-mediated immune responses. This drug is associated with the risk of lymphoma in some patients. Other side effects of azathioprine include bone marrow suppression and vomiting.

***Mercaptopurine*** is a structural analog of guanine that leads to disruption in purine synthesis and inhibition of DNA and RNA synthesis. In addition to a treatment for IBD, it is also used in acute lymphocytic leukemia and chronic myeloid leukemia.

***Methotrexate*** acts through the inhibition of enzymes involved in purine metabolism. This leads to the inhibition of T-lymphocyte and B-lymphocyte activation. Another proposed mechanism of methotrexate is its ability to inhibit the binding of interleukin-1 to surface receptors and prevent the activation of an inflammatory response. Methotrexate can lead to bone marrow suppression and an increase in infection risk.

## Antibiotics

Although ***metronidazole*** and other antibiotics do not play a role in suppressing the immune response that causes IBD, incorporating them into the treatment regime may help prevent gastrointestinal complications like abscess formation, postoperative infections, and overgrowth of microorganisms in the gut.

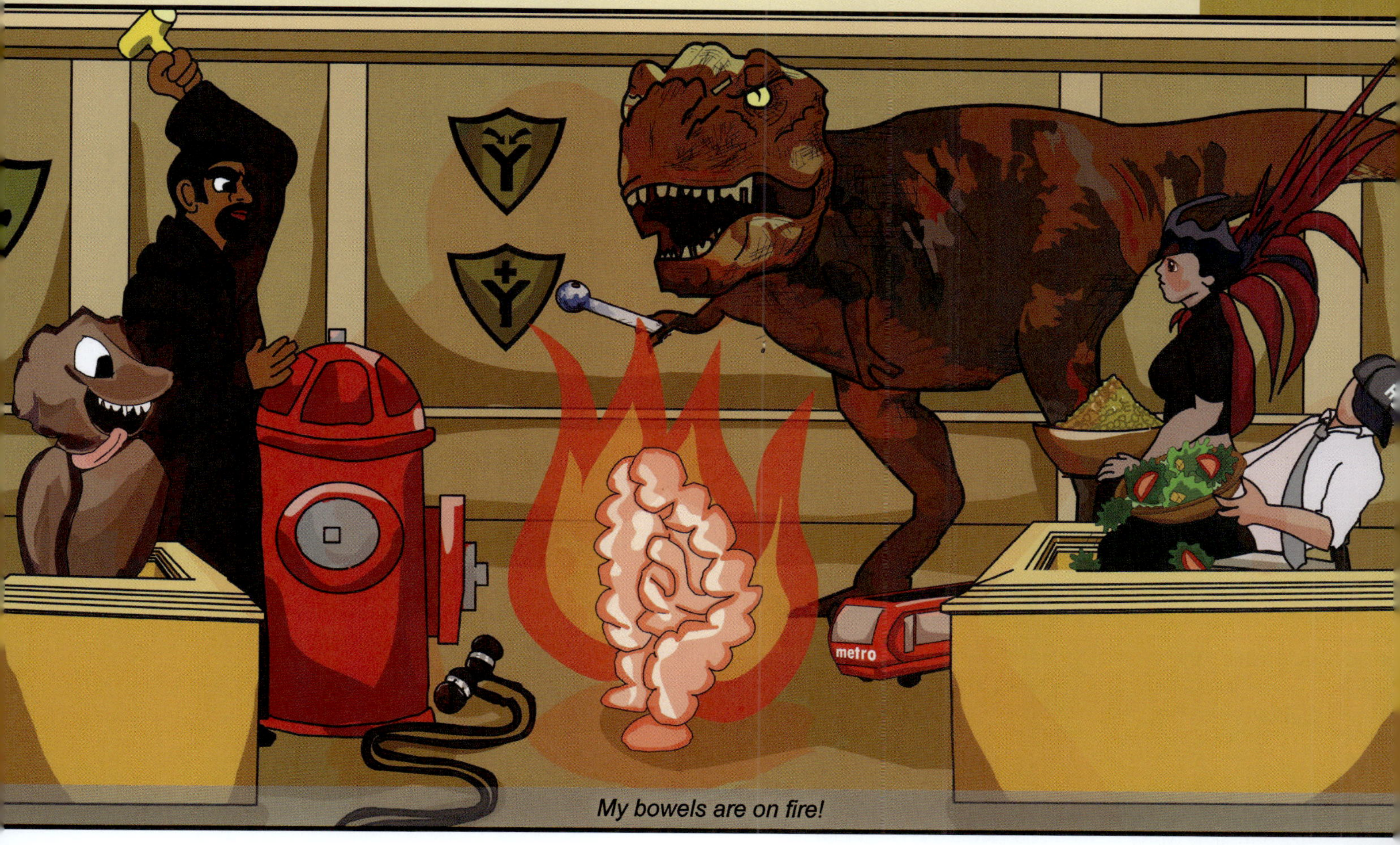


## INFLAMMATORY BOWEL DISEASE

*The bowel on fire reminds you this picture is about inflammatory bowel disease!*

### Corticosteroids

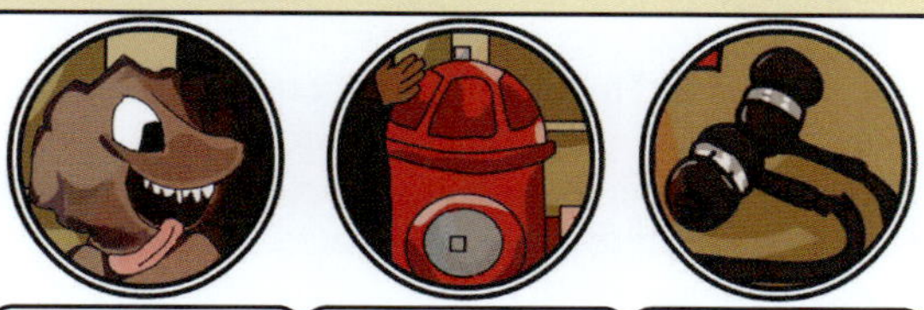

| "Predator" | "Hydro-Court" | "[Ear]-Buds" |
|---|---|---|
| **Prednisolone** | **Hydrocortisone** | **Budesonide** |

### Aminosalicylates

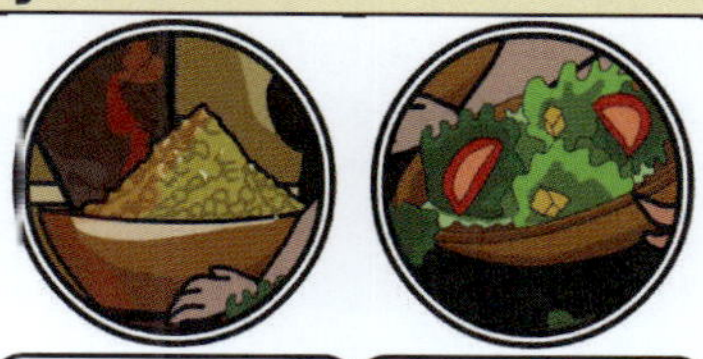

| "Sulfur-Salad" | "Messy-Salad" |
|---|---|
| **Sulfasalazine** | **Mesalazine** |

### Monoclonal Antibodies

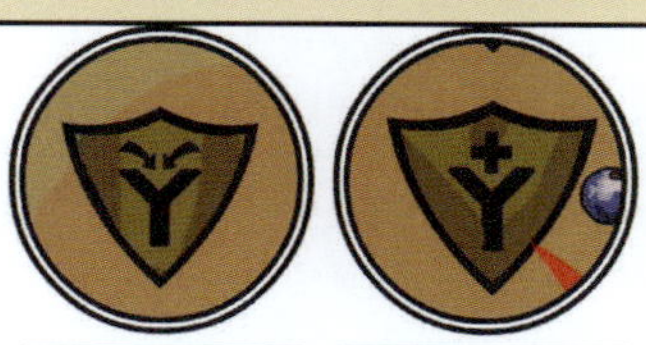

| "Influx-mAb" | "Add-mAb" |
|---|---|
| **Infliximab** | **Adalimumab** |

### Mucosal Protectants

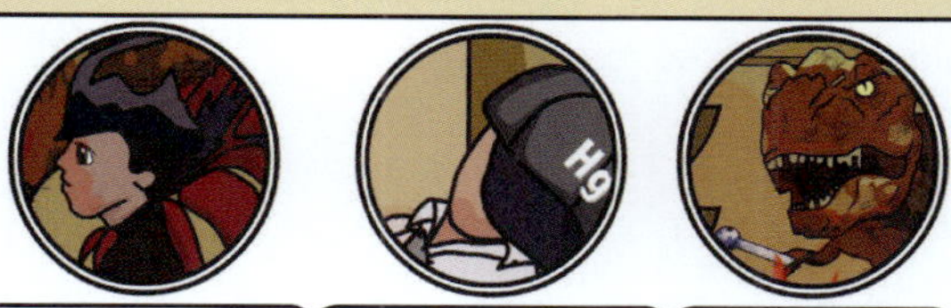


| "Aztek-Princess" | "Mercury-Cap" | "Meth-T-Rex" |
|---|---|---|
| **Azathioprine** | **Mercaptopurine** [Mercury is Hg on periodic table] | **Methotrexate** |

### Antibiotics

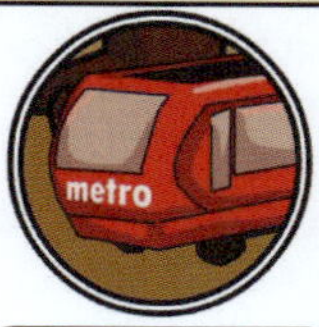


| "Metro" |
|---|
| **Metronidazole** |

# LAXATIVES AND ANTIDIARRHOEALS DISEASE

**Indications for laxatives:** constipation.
**Indications for antidiarrhoeals:** diarrhoea.

**DIARRHEA AND CONSTIPATION** are changes in bowel habits that can often impact people's quality of life. Diarrhea is an increase in frequency of bowel movements in a liquid form. Constipation is a decrease in frequency of bowel movements, characterized by passing hard stools, straining, and painful bowel movements. Bowel habits can be influenced by factors such as diet, stress, neuromuscular disorders of the gastrointestinal tract, endocrine disorders, and cancer. Medication and hydration therapy are often used at treatment.

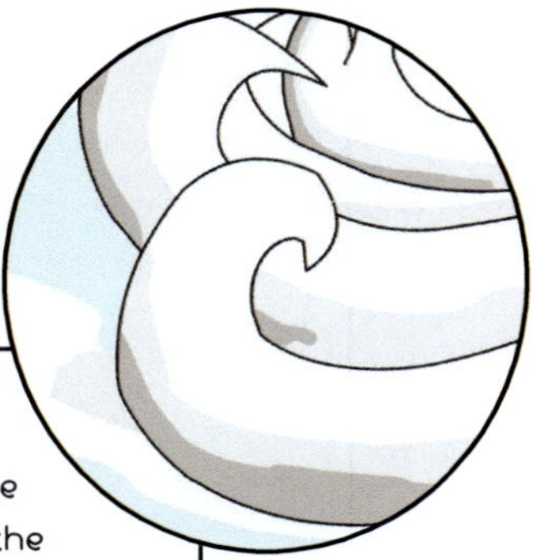

The laxative drugs have caused a tidal wave of bowel motions, while the antidiorrhoeals are on the top right of the picture.

## Laxatives

Constipation is usually treated with laxatives. Laxatives can be classified into ***bulk forming, osmotic, stimulant, motility stimulant***, and ***softener*** laxatives.

### Bulk-Forming

Bulk laxatives laxatives are often first line agents for constipation. Their consumption should be accompanied with adequate water intake to prevent intestinal obstruction.

Bulk-forming laxatives, like ***bran*** or ***ispaghula***, promote water absorption in the colon to increase the bulk of fecal matter and distention of the bowel. This initiates a reflex in bowel activity and eases the passing of stools out of the body.

### Osmotic

Osmotic laxatives, including ***lactulose*** and ***magnesium sulfate***, are poorly absorbed in the intestines and thereby promote water retention by osmosis into the bowel. As a result, soft and bulky stools are formed and distention of gut wall occurs leading to stimulation of bowel movements.

### Stimulant

Stimulant laxatives directly stimulate the enteric nervous system and promote colonic electrolyte and fluid secretion by increasing prostaglandin and cAMP levels. Some examples of stimulant laxatives are ***senna***, ***bisacodyl***, and ***docusate***. Stimulant laxatives are extremely powerful and should only be used for a short term.

### Motility Stimulant

Motility stimulant laxatives, such as ***metoclopramide*** or ***domperidone***, are conventionally used to prevent nausea and vomiting and for treating delayed stomach emptying. These drugs are also effective for constipation due to their ability to stimulate bowel activity through binding to dopamine-D2 receptors in the small intestine.

### Faecal Softeners

Faecal softeners, such as ***liquid paraffin***, are used to soften the stool to make it easier to pass. Liquid Paraffin is a mineral oil that nowadays is not recommended, as it can seep from anus and lead to irritation.

## Antidiarrhoeals

Diarrhea is usually managed using opiates and their derivatives. These drugs include ***loperamide***, ***codeine*** or ***morphine***.

***Loperamide*** is a spasmolytic agent often used to suppress diarrhea in diseases such as gastroenteritis, inflammatory bowel disease (IBD), or short bowel syndrome. Pharmacologically, loperamide is an opioid agonist and it acts directly on mu-receptors located in the myenteric plexus of the large intestines. This leads to a decrease in activity of the myenteric plexus, and an overall decrease in tone of the smooth muscles in the intestinal wall responsible for movement of material through the GI tract. If the clinical picture leads to the suspicion of an infection caused by microorganisms that can potentially penetrate the colon lining, loperamide is contraindicated as a first line agent to prevent exacerbation. Other severe side effects of this drug include toxic megacolon, paralytic ileus, toxic epidermal necrolysis and Stevens-Johnson syndrome.

***Codeine*** binds to opioid receptors on the walls of the intestines, and thereby decreasing peristalsis. This leads to more time for water and minerals to be absorbed in the intestine.

***Morphine*** is rarely used to treat diarrhea nowaday due to its addictive properties, however, in certain circumstances can be a powerful treatment option. Like loperamide and codeine, it acts on opioid receptors to decrease peristalsis.

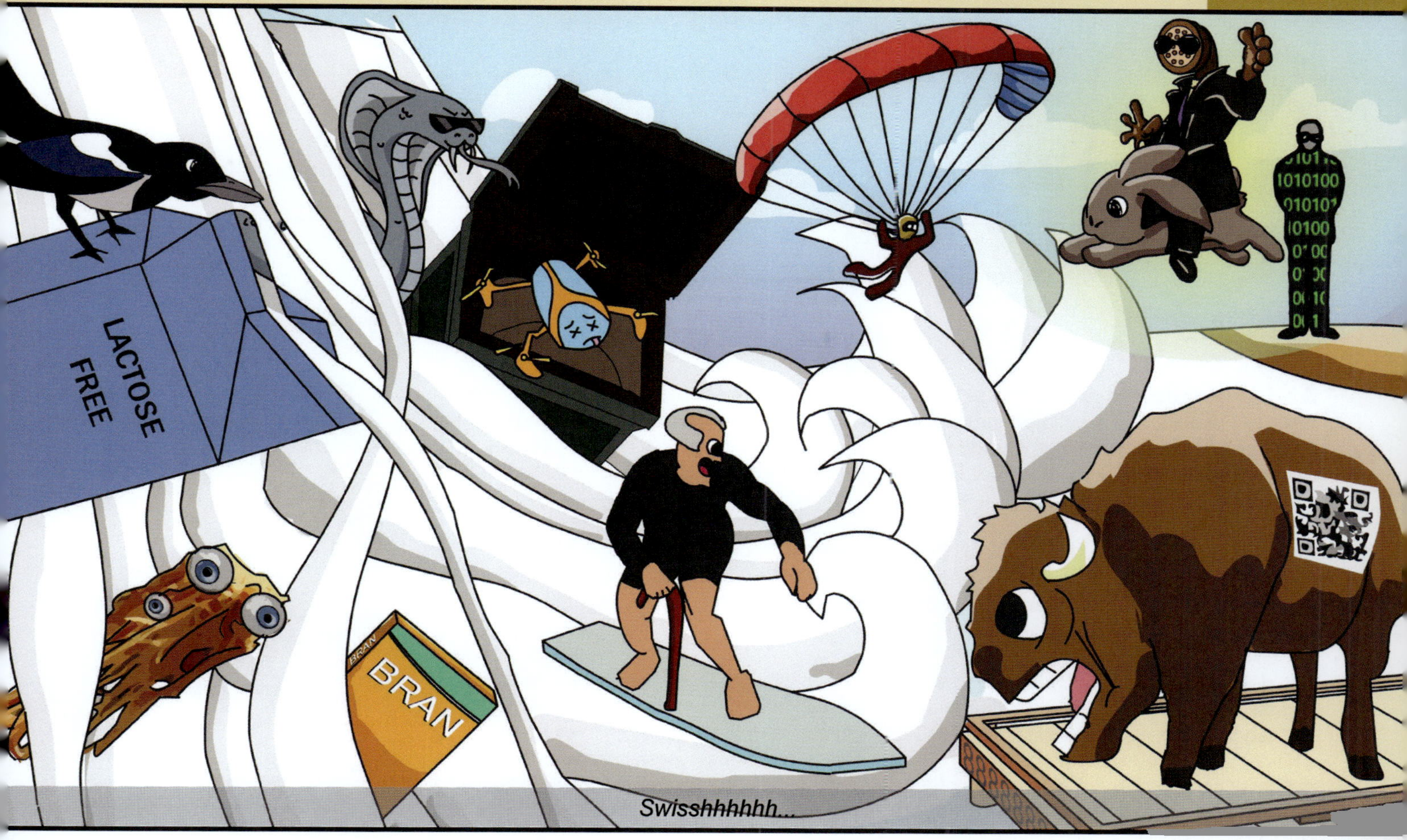


## LAXATIVES AND ANTIDIARRHOEALS

*The laxative drugs have caused a tidal wave of bowel motions, while the antidiorrhoeals are on the top right of the picture.*

### Bulk Forming Laxatives

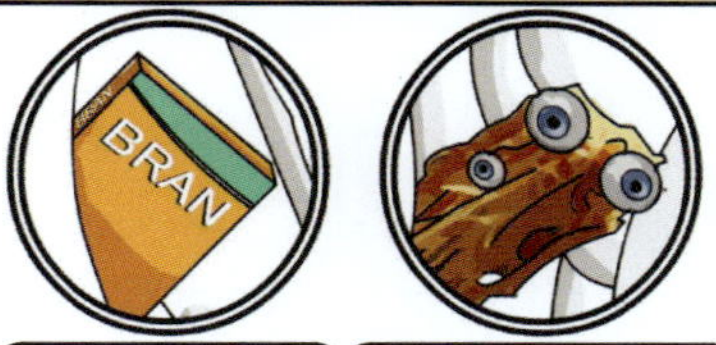


*"Bran"* **Bran**

*"Eye-Spaghetti"* **Ispaghula**

### Osmotic Laxatives

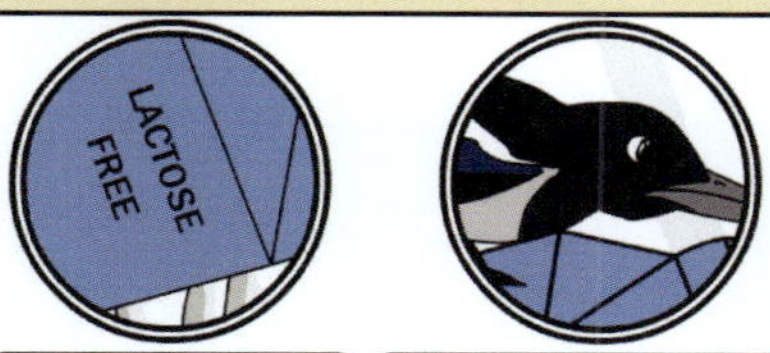


*"Lactose-[free]"* **Lactulose**

*"Magpie"* **Magnesium Sulfate**

### Stimulant Laxatives

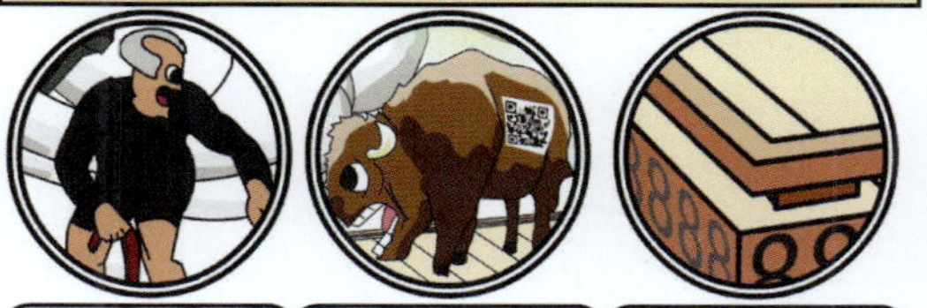

*"Senior"* **Senna**

*"Bison-Code"* **Bisacodyl**

*"Dock-Eight"* **Docusate**

### Motility Stimulants Laxatives

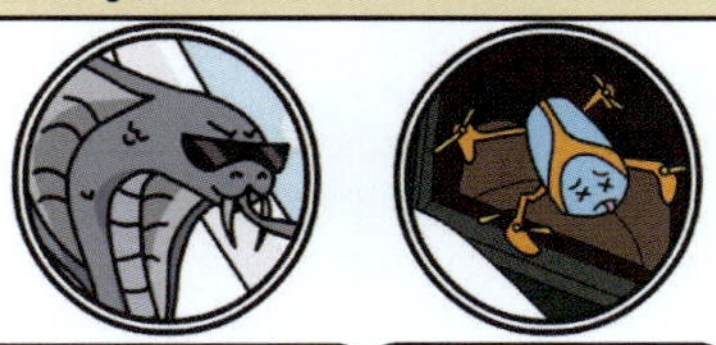

*"Metal-Cobra"* **Metoclopramide**

*"Dump-Drone"* **Domperidone**

### Softener Laxatives

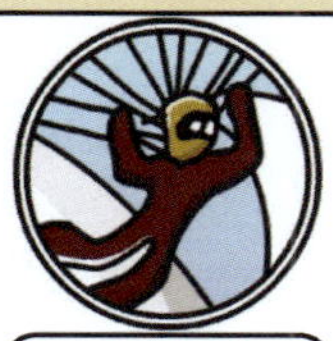

*"Parachute"* **Paraffin**

### Antidiarrhoeals

*"Lop-Ear"* **Loperamide**

*"Code-Being"* **Codeine**

*"Morpheus-Phone"* **Morphine**

# ANEMIA

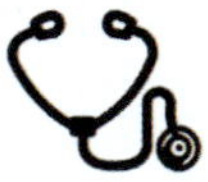

**Indications for anemia medications:** iron deficiency anemia.

**ANEMIA** is defined as a decrease in haemoglobin concentration, hematocrit, or red blood cell (RBC) count. The function of red blood cells is to transport oxygen from the lungs to the peripheral tissues and carbon dioxide from the tissues to the lungs. Therefore, gaseous exchange processes in the body will be greatly impaired when red blood cell volumes are reduced.

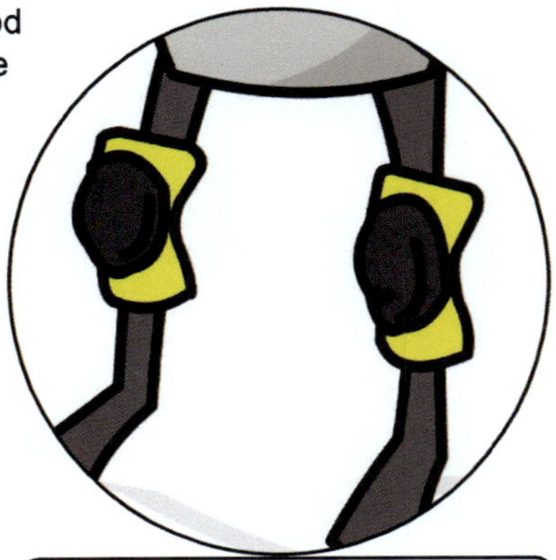

The knee-pads on each character remind you this picture is about anemia (a-knee-mia).

Pathophysiology of anemia can be explained by several mechanisms including blood loss, decreases in RBC production, and increases in RBC destruction. Investigations to determine the underlying cause is essential, as the etiology will guide management of the anemia.

Iron deficiency anemia is caused by low iron levels, which is usually due to blood loss, but can also be due to poor dietary intake or decreased absorption. Low iron levels will cause your body to make fewer and smaller RBCs, which can lead to deficiencies in oxygen delivery. Some causes of blood loss include trauma, ulcers, heavy periods, or colon cancer. Decreased absorption of iron can occur from conditions such as Crohn's disease or gastric bypass.

Anemias caused by decreases in RBC production are likely due to folic acid or vitamin B12 deficiency, and lead to megaloblastic anemia; however, it can also be caused by bone marrow disorders, such as aplastic anemia; bone marrow suppression, such as can occur on chemotherapy; disorders such as alpha and beta thalassemia; myelodysplastic syndrome; and sideroblastic anemia.

Increases in RBC destruction may be due to trauma, or an inherited or acquired RBC disorder. Examples of inherited disorders include, sickle cell disease, thalassemia major, and hereditary spherocytosis. Examples of acquired RBC disorders include secondary thrombotic thrombocytopenic purpura and malaria.

## Iron Preparations

Iron deficiency anemia is treated with ***iron*** supplementation therapy. Iron can be taken orally in the form of iron preparations, such as ***iron dextran*** or ***sucrose***; or ferrous preparations, such as ***ferrous sulphate, gluconate***, or ***fumarate***. Iron administration should be carried out with caution as excessive iron intake can be toxic and lead to accumulation of iron in the body, ultimately damaging organs.

## Folic Acid

Folic acid deficiency is usually caused by low dietary intake and is treated with ***folic acid*** supplementation. Folic acid is required for the synthesis of DNA which allows cells to divide. Therefore, its deficiency impairs the ability of RBCs to proceed through the cell cycle, and as a result, the RBC will appear to be abnormally large in size under the microscope, which is an indication of immature and dysfunctional RBC.

## Vitamin B12

***Vitamin B12*** is also needed to make healthy RBCs. Vitamin B12 deficiency is often caused by pernicious anemia, an autoimmune condition that leads to loss of parietal cells in the stomach required to make intrinsic factor. Intrinsic factor binds to Vitamin B12, and is required for its absorption in the intestine. Vitamin B12 deficiency can also occur due to lack of dietary intake, various conditions that affect the stomach and intestine such as Crohn's disease, and is associated with chronic alcoholism.

## Treatment for Iron Overdose

***Deferoxamine*** is a medication that binds iron in blood and causes increased iron release in the urine. It is used for treatment of iron overdose and haemochromatosis.

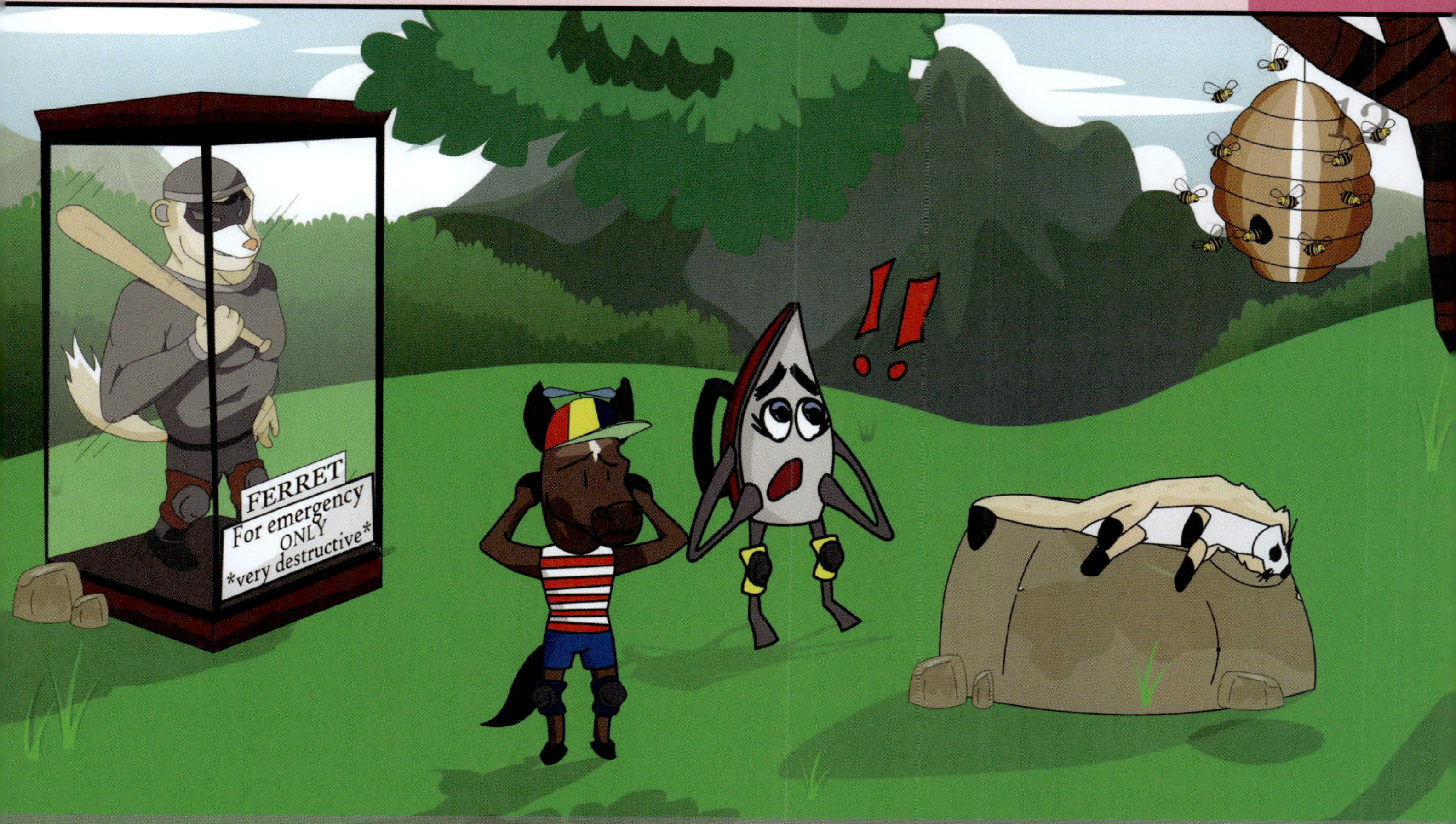


*An anemic ferret in danger!*

## ANEMIA

☞ *The knee-pads on each character remind you this picture is about anemia (a-knee-mia).*

### Iron Preparations

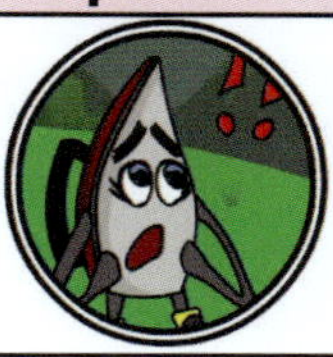

*"Iron"*
**Iron**
[dextran or sucrose]

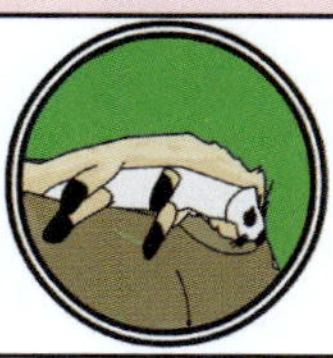

*"Ferret"*
**Ferrous**
[sulphate, gluconate or fumerate]

### Folic Acid

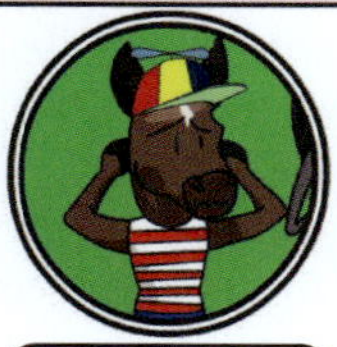

*"Foal"*
**Folic acid**

### Vitamin $B_{12}$

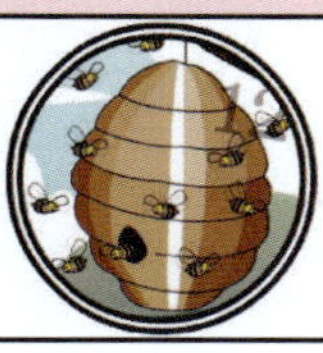

*"12-Bees"*
**Vitamin B12**
[hydroxycobalamin]

### Treatment for Iron Overdose

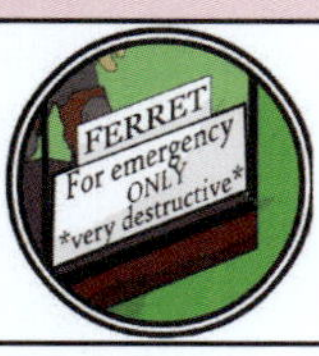


*"Destructive-Ferret"*
**Deferoxamine**

# ANTICOAGULANTS

**Indications for anticoagulant medications:** atrial fibrillation, mechanical heart valves, VTE, MI, acute ischaemic stroke.

**IN MEDICINE, COAGULATION** is defined as a physiological process in which blood is converted from liquid to a semi-solid or solid state, forming a thrombus. According to Virchow's Triad, blood coagulation is affected by three factors: **endothelial wall damage**, **stagnation of blood**, and a **hypercoagulable state**.

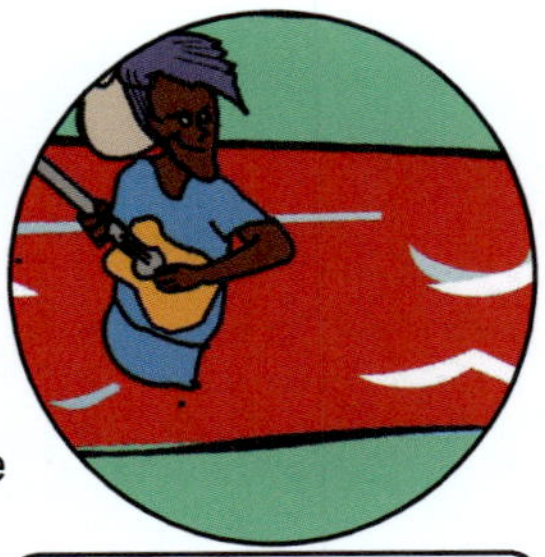

The red river is like a blood stream, which is blocked by the guitarists. This reminds you of coagulation!

While thrombosis itself is a compensatory mechanism to prevent excessive blood loss, an abnormal increase of thrombus formation may lead to life threatening pulmonary embolism, stroke, and acute coronary syndrome. Patients who have developed complications related to hypercoagulability or those at high risk need to be on anticoagulant therapy (commonly known as blood thinners).

## Vitamin K Antagonists

***Warfarin*** is the classic representation of a blood thinner, and is used in treatment of deep vein thrombosis and pulmonary emboli. It is used to prevent stroke in those who are at high risk, such as those with atrial fibrillation, who have an artificial heart valve, or have valvular heart disease.

Warfarin acts as a vitamin K antagonist which inhibits the synthesis of clotting factors in the liver. It does so by inhibiting an enzyme called vitamin K reductase, an enzyme required for clotting factor activation using vitamin K. The clotting factors in which warfarin inhibits are factor II, VII, IX, and X. It is usually taken orally, but in some cases may be administered intravenously.

The common adverse effect of warfarin is bleeding, but it can be reversed with the administration of vitamin K or fresh frozen plasma (FFP) and is monitored through a blood test measuring international normalized ratio (INR). A few days may be required for warfarin to reach its full efficacy and its effects may last up to 5 days.

## Heparins

***Unfractionated heparin*** is a type of blood thinner that prevents the formation of thrombi in the body. Like warfarin, it is mainly used for the treatment of deep vein thrombosis and pulmonary embolism, however, it has a different mechanism of action.

Unfractionated heparin binds to a small protein molecule called antithrombin III, leading to a change in its structural configuration and the inactivation of factor Xa and thrombin, which are involved in the coagulation cascade that ultimately causes fibrin needed for blood clotting. Heparin can lead to a major side effect known as heparin induced thrombocytopenia (HIT). This is an immunological response that targets the platelets and can result in massive bleeding due to low platelet count. In the case of overdose or circumstances that require the reversion of heparin effect, protamine sulfate can be used as an antidote.

## Low Molecular Weight Heparin (LMWH)

There is another variant of anticoagulant that resembles heparin called ***low molecular weight heparins*** (***LMWHs***). These anticoagulants inhibit factor Xa to a greater extent than heparin. LMWHs have a greater bioavailability, a longer half life, and a more predictable anticoagulant response than unfractionated heparin. LMWHs are typically administered subcutaneously, and its use does not require the monitoring of a patient's coagulation profile like warfarin.

LMWHs are contraindicated in patients with end stage kidney failure due to the route of its metabolism. Patients with a history of a LMWH allergy or those who have experienced HIT should also avoid taking this drug. Examples of LMWH are ***fondaparinux***, ***enoxaparin,*** and ***dalteparin***.

## Direct Factor Xa inhibitors

Direct factor Xa inhibitors, such as ***rivaroxaban*** and ***apixaban***, are medications that inhibit factor Xa, an enzyme of the coagulation cascade that converts prothrombin to thrombin. This enzyme is needed for the conversion of fibrinogen to fibrin in the formation of blood clots. Although direct factor Xa inhibitors are associated with a lower risk of fatal bleeding, they have been shown to increase the chance of gastrointestinal bleeding when compared to traditional blood thinners like warfarin and heparin.

## Direct Thrombin Inhibitors

Direct thrombin inhibitors, such as ***dabigatran***, are effective for the prevention of stroke and atrial fibrillation not caused by prosthetic heart valves. This class of drug should be avoided in patients who have active bleeding and those with the history of hypersensitivity reaction such as anaphylactic shock.

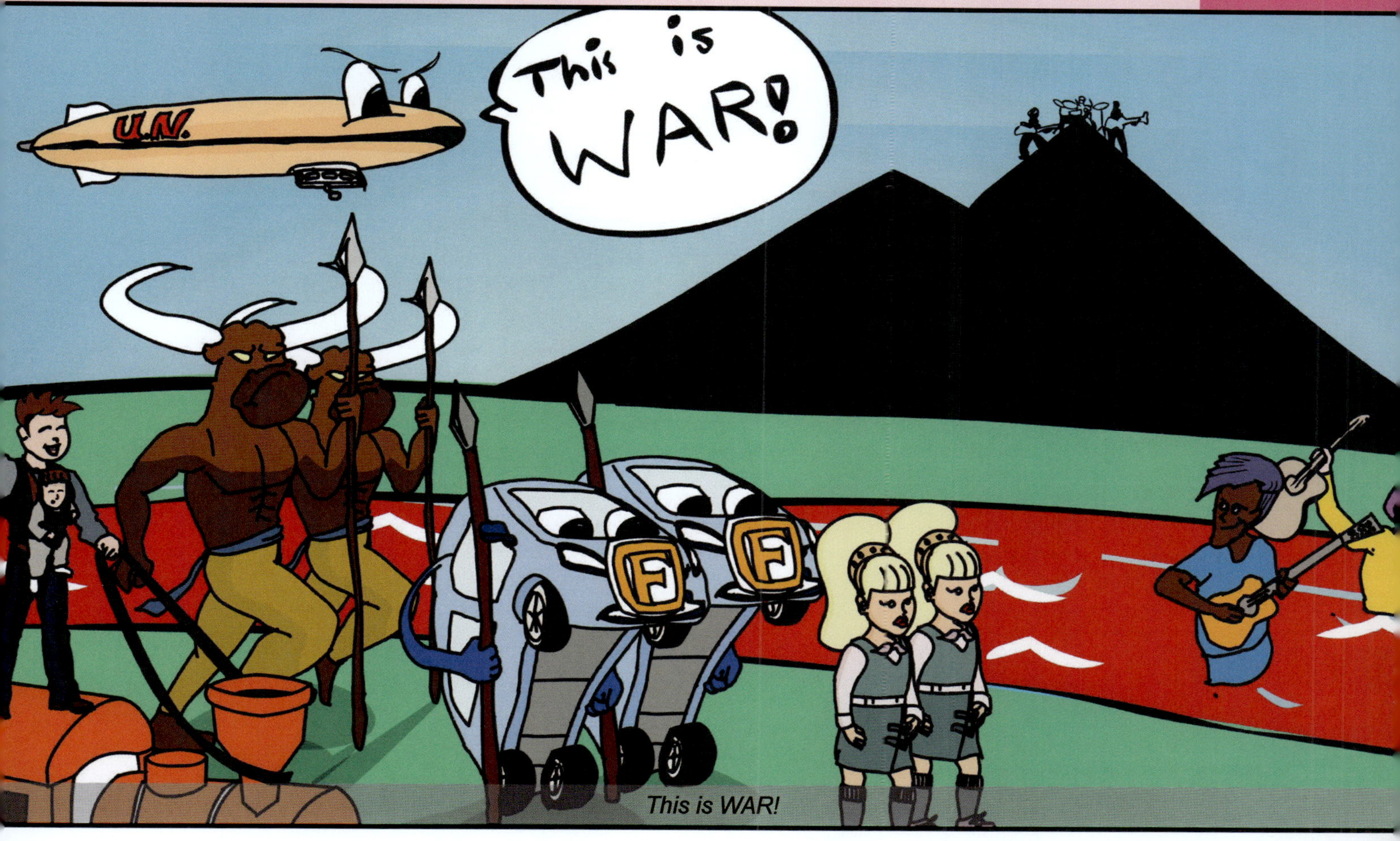

This is WAR!

### ANTICOAGULANTS

*The red river is like a blood stream, which is blocked by the guitarists. This reminds you of coagulation!*

#### Vitamin K Antagonists

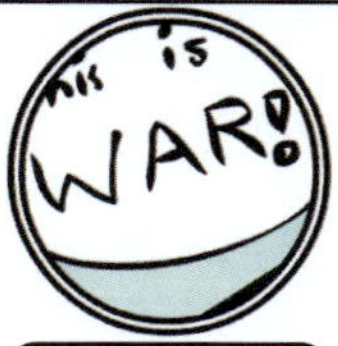


*"War"*
**Warfarin**

#### Heparins

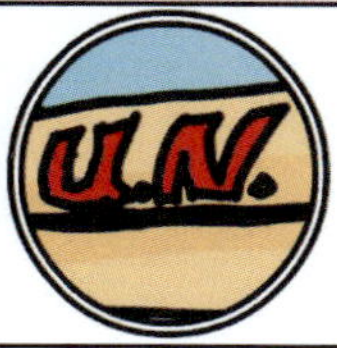


*"U.N.-Zeppelin"*
**Unfractionated Heparin**

#### LMWH

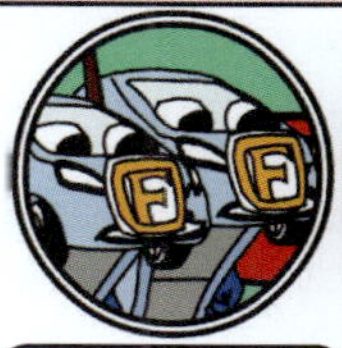

*"Fonda-Pair"*
**Fondaparinux**

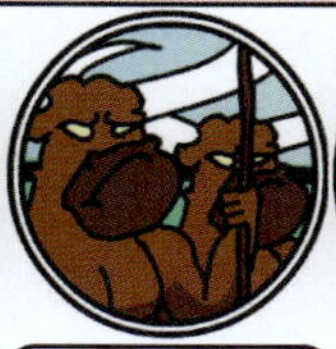

*"Ox-Pair"*
**Enoxaparin**

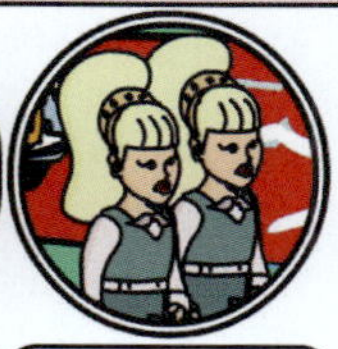

*"Doll-Pair"*
**Dalteparin**

#### Direct Factor Xa Inhibitor

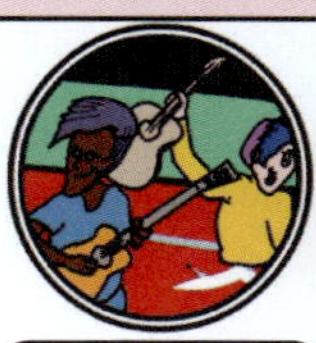

*"River-Band"*
**Rivaroxaban**

*"Apex-Band"*
**Apixaban**

#### Direct Thrombin Inhibitor

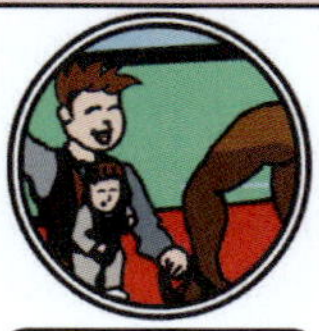

*"Dad-Train"*
**Dabigatran**

# ANTIPLATELETS AND FIBRINOLYTICS

**Indications for antiplatelet medications:** CAD, ischemic stroke, MI, atrial fibrillation.
**Indications for fibrinolytic medications:** acute MI, ischemic stroke, PE, DVT.

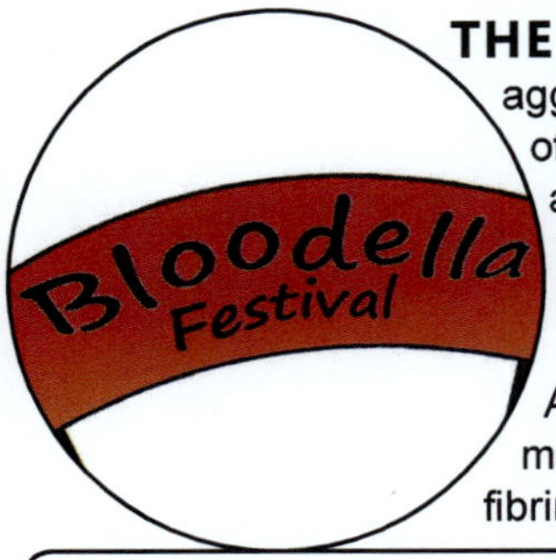


**THE ANTIPLATELET DRUGS** are a class of medication used for the prevention of platelet aggregation in arterial thrombosis. Platelets only become activated when the endothelial wall of a blood vessel becomes damaged leading to the stimulation of chemical substances such as collagen, thromboxane A2, adenosine diphosphate (ADP), and thrombin. This hemostatic process is particularly significant as it is the main pathophysiology behind life-threatening medical conditions such as myocardial infarction and stroke.

Antiplatelet drugs play a large role in preventing clustered platelets from occluding the patency of major blood vessels. In clinical conditions where a thrombus is already occluding a blood vessel, fibrinolytics can used to break down the thrombus and restore patency of the vasculature.

Bloodella is a play on Coachella festival. The blood component reminds you the picture is about antiplatelets and fibrinolytics!

## COX Inhibitors

The most commonly used antiplatelet agent is ***aspirin***. Classified as a cyclooxygenase (COX) inhibitor, aspirin is widely known for its analgesic function due to its ability to inhibit pain mediators such as prostaglandin E2 (PGE2). Inhibition of COX also prevents the formation of other chemical substances that lead to platelets aggregation, including thromboxane A2 and prostaglandin D2 (PGD2). Aspirin remains a first line treatment for prevention of myocardial infarction and stroke.

## Adenosine Diphosphate (ADP) Receptor Inhibitors

***Clopidogrel*** and ***ticagrelor*** are examples of ADP receptor inhibitors. Similar to aspirin, they are capable of stopping platelet aggregation and are used for the prevention of myocardial infarction and stroke. They work by inhibiting ADP receptors found on the surface of platelet cell membranes, which are important for the activation of platelet aggregation and subsequently the cross-linking process of fibrin formation. Since ADP receptor inhibitors work through a different mechanism of action than aspirin, they are suitable for cardiac patients who cannot tolerate aspirin.

## Glycoprotein (Gp) IIb/IIIa inhibitors

***Tirofiban*** and ***abciximab*** can be used to prevent the formation of platelet aggregation during cardiac events. They are also used before percutaneous coronary intervention like angioplasty to prevent thrombus formation. GpIIb/IIIa receptors are found on the surface of platelets and mediate chemical interactions between platelets and other ligands (e.g. fibrinogen). GpIIb/IIIa inhibitors antagonize these receptors to prevent the aggregation of platelets. Side effects include bleeding and hypersensitivity.

## Adenosine Reuptake Inhibitors

Adenosine reuptake inhibitors, such as ***dipyridamole***, are drugs that act by inhibiting phosphodiesterase, and in turn, block the platelet aggregation response to ADP. As its name suggests, it also prevents the reuptake of adenosine into platelets and thereby increase extracellular levels of adenosine.

## Fibrinolytics

As mentioned earlier, platelet aggregation and thrombus formation can be reversed with the use of fibrinolytics. These drugs are usually administered intravenously during emergency thrombotic events such as pulmonary embolism and ischaemic stroke.

***Streptokinase***, ***alteplase,*** and ***reteplase*** are examples of fibrinolytics. These agents are able to form an active complex with plasminogen. This complex will activate plasmin to facilitate the breakdown of fibrin into soluble degradation products in the bloodstream. Similar to other antiplatelet agents, fibrinolytics increase the chances of serious bleeding and therefore, the coagulation profile of the patients must be checked thoroughly before administration of these drugs.

## Antifibrinolytics

Antifibrinolytics such as ***tranexamic acid*** (***TXA***) bind reversibly to the receptor sites of plasminogen. As a result, it prevents the binding action of plasminogen to fibrin to maintain the framework of fibrin in the site of injury. It is commonly administered intravenously in clinical practice for the prevention of major blood loss during trauma or postpartum bleeding.

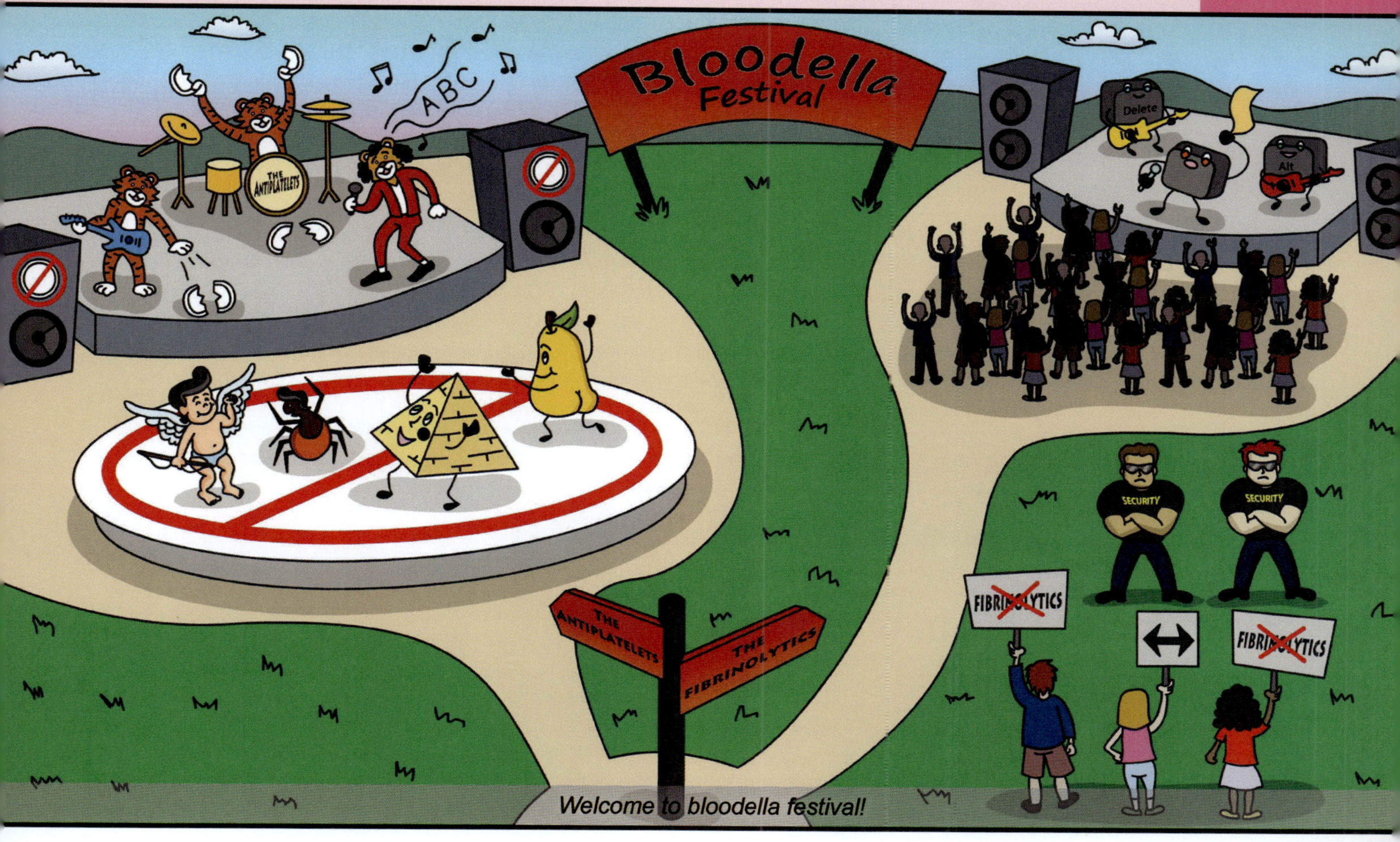


## ANTIPLATELETS AND FIBRINOLYTICS

*Bloodella is a play on Coachella festival. The blood component reminds you the picture is about antiplatelets and fibrinolytics!*

### COX Inhibitors

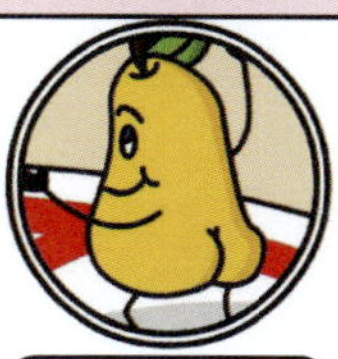

*"Ass-Pear"*
**Aspirin**

### ADP Receptor Inhibitors

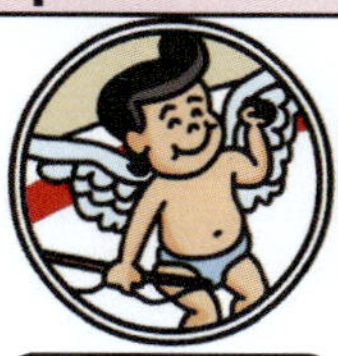

*"Cupid"*
**Clopidogrel**

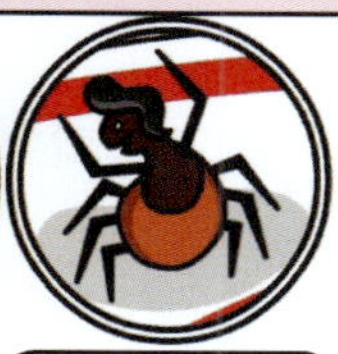

*"Tick-Gel"*
**Ticagrelor**

### GP IIB/IIIA Inhibitors

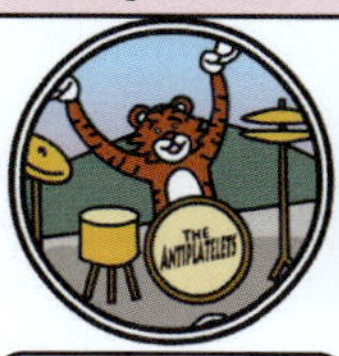


*"Tiger-Band"*
**Tirofiban**

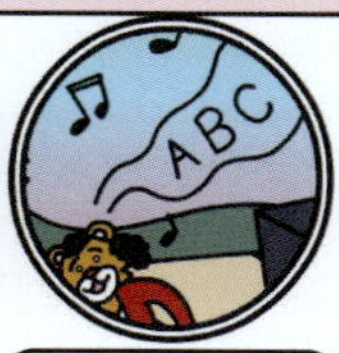


*"ABC"*
**Abciximab**

### Adenosine Reuptake Inhibitor

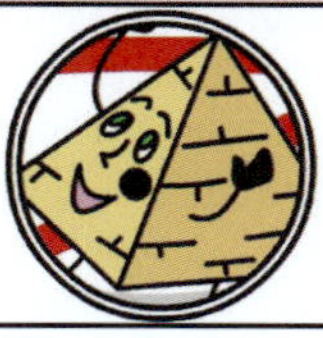

*"Pyramid-Mole"*
**Dipyridamole**

### Fibrinolytic Drugs

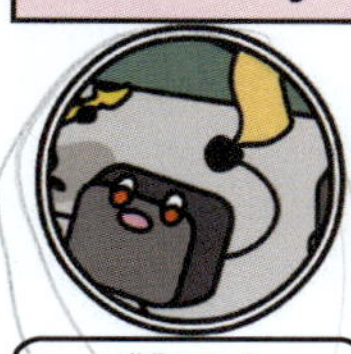

*"Strip"*
**Streptokinase**

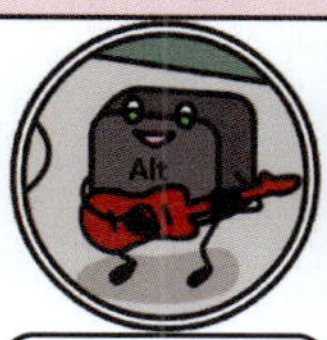


*"Alt"*
**Alteplase**

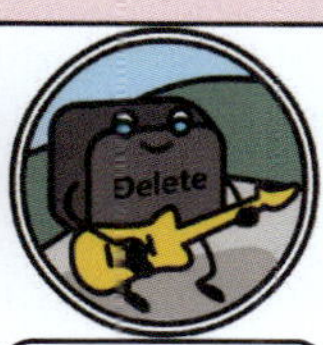


*"Delete"*
**Reteplase**

### Antifibrinolytic Drugs

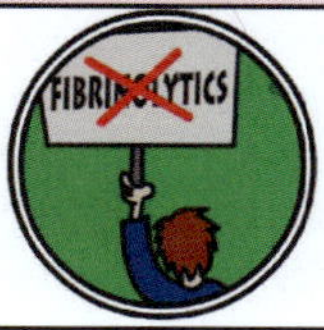


*"X"*
**Tranexamic Acid**

# ANTIBACTERIAL DRUGS: INHIBIT CELL WALL SYNTHESIS

**Indications for antibacterial medications:** bacterial infections (UTIs, URTIs, LRTIs, sepsis, skin infections, etc), prophylaxis in patients with compromised immune systems.

**MANY ANTIBIOTICS** produce their effects by targeting cell walls of bacteria. These medications are widely prescribed and are very effective. Specifically, they function by binding to penicillin binding proteins, thereby preventing formation of cross links in the bacterial peptidoglycan cell wall. As a result, the increased osmotic gradient between the inside and outside of the cell wall leads to leakage and degradation of the cell content. Some bacteria evolve over time and are able to counter the effect of these types of antibiotics through the production of beta-lactamase, which breaks down the beta-lactam ring structure in these drugs. In this case, beta-lactamase resistant antibiotics can be used.

The most common types of antibiotics that target cell wall synthesis are penicillins and cephalosporins. Penicillins can be split into narrow spectrum, broad spectrum, and antipseudomonal classes, and are effective against gram positive bacteria. Cephalosporins typically target gram positive bacteria, however, do vary in their ability to treat gram negative infections.

## Narrow Spectrum Penicillins

An example of a narrow-spectrum penicillin is ***benzylpenicillin***, which is effective against gram positive bacteria such as Staphylococci and Streptococci. This medication is often used for strep throat and syphilis.

***Flucloxacillin*** is another commonly used narrow spectrum antibiotic that has beta-lactamase resistance, and therefore can be used to treat beta-lactamases producing organisms. Most commonly, it is used to treat chest, skin, ear, nose, and throat infections.

## Broad Spectrum Penicillins

By definition, broad-spectrum penicillins are effective against a wide range of bacteria. Examples include ***amoxicillin*** and ***ampicillin***. They are used for the treatment of otitis media, sore throat, pneumonia or urinary tract infection.

## Antipseudomonal Penicillins

***Piperacillin*** and ***ticarcillin*** are beta-lactamase penicillin antibiotics that contain antipseudomonal properties. These antibiotics are for patients infected with gram negative bacteria, particularly rod-shaped bacteria called Pseudomonas aeruginosa. Piperacillin is often used in combination with a beta-lactamase inhibitor, such as tazobactam, to treat severe hospital-acquired infections like pneumonia. Ticarcillin is also often used in combination with a beta lactamase inhibitor such as clavulanic acid, and is used to treat a variety of infections which include: urinary tract infections, bone and joint infections, and skin infections.

## Cephalosporins

There are four generations of cephalosporins, with each generation having different clinical efficacy against specific types of bacteria. First generation cephalosporins such as ***cephalexin***, are effective predominantly against gram positive bacteria.

***Cefuroxime*** is a second generation cephalosporin, and it has great efficacy against Haemophilus influenzae, Neisseria gonorrhoeae and Lyme disease. Unlike most other second generation cephalosporins, cefuroxime is able to cross the blood brain barrier and therefore, can be used to treat meningitis.

***Ceftriaxone*** and ***ceftazidime*** are third generation cephalosporins. Ceftriaxone is widely used due to its efficacy against many bacterial strains including those that are antibiotic resistant. However, it is not effective against Pseudomonas aeruginosa and Enterobacter infections.

The fourth generation cephalosporin are the newest class, of which examples include ***cefepime*** and ***cefpirome***. They cover an extended spectrum of activity against gram-positive and gram-negative bacteria, more so than third generation cephalosporins.

## Others

***Meropenem*** and ***aztreonam*** are both beta-lactam antibiotics, so their mode of action is similar to penicillins and cephalosporins. Meropenem is usually reserved for the treatment of infections caused by multi-drug resistant bacteria. Therefore, they are only used in severe cases and in hospital acquired bacterial infections such as pneumonia and severe sepsis. Aztreonam is primarily used to treat gram negative infections, including being able to treat pseudomonal infections.

***Vancomycin*** is the most effective drug treatment for methicillin resistant staphylococcus aureus (MRSA) infections. Infection by MRSA usually occurs in patients who are in a healthcare setting for an extended period of time, and is closely associated with invasive procedures such as surgeries, intravenous tube insertions, or joint prosthesis fixation.

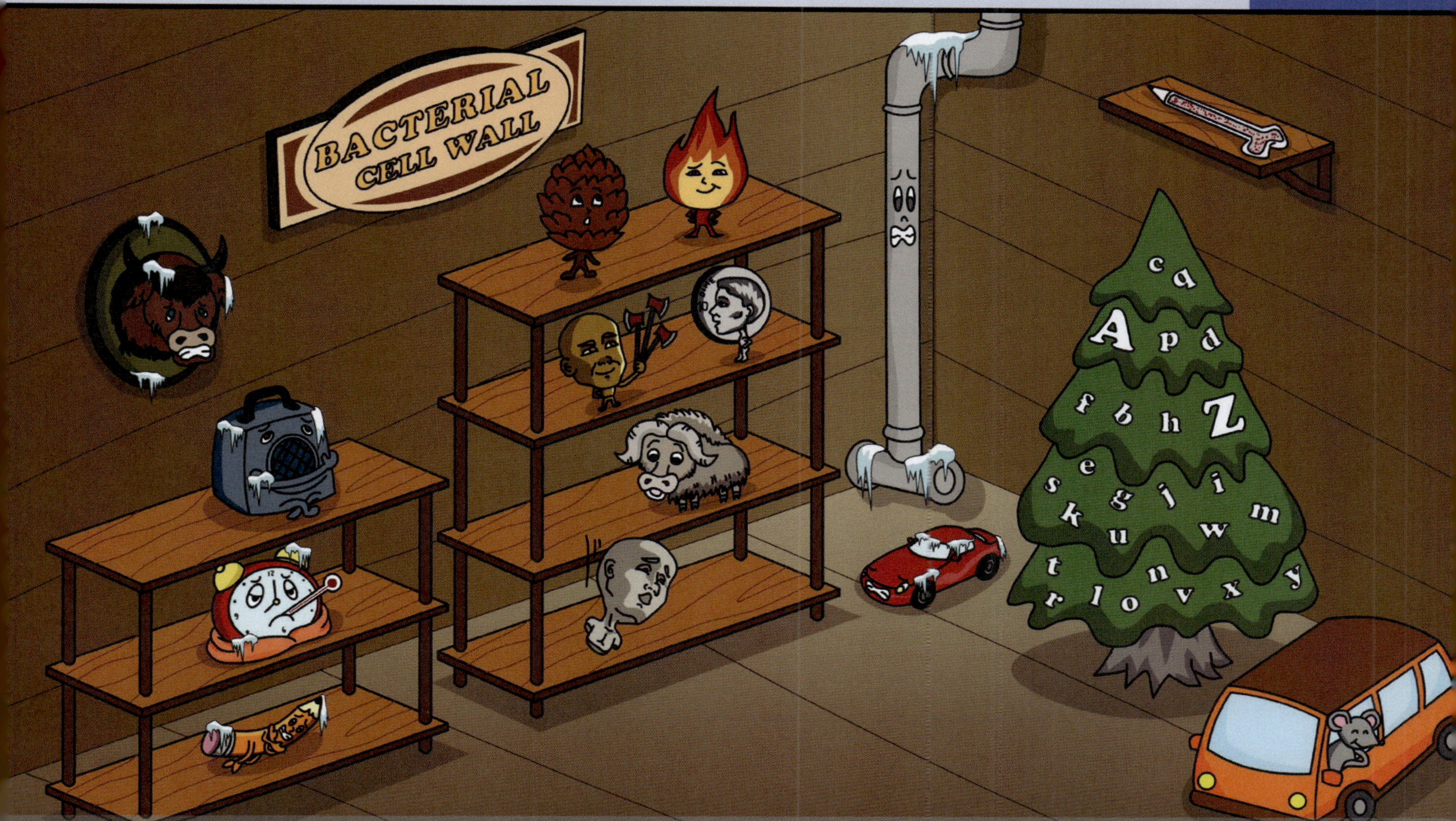


*What a wall!*

## ANTIBACTERIAL DRUGS THAT INHIBIT CELL WALL SYNTHESIS

☞ *The sign "bacterial cell wall" reminds you this picture is about antibiotics that target cell walls.*

### Penicillins - Narrow

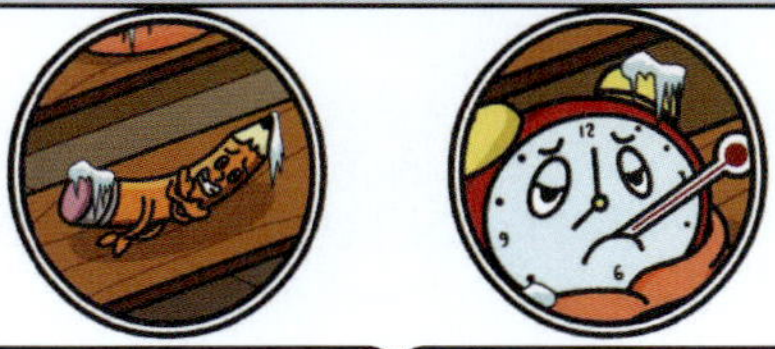

*"Bent-Pencil-Chilling"* **Benzylpenicillin**

*"Flu-Clock-Chilling"* **Flucloxacillin**

### Penicillins - Broad

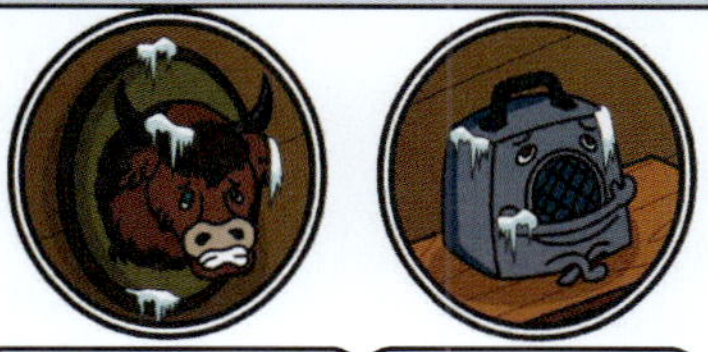

*"An-Ox-Chilling"* **Amoxicillin**

*"Amp-Chilling"* **Ampicillin**

### Antipseudomonal Penicillins

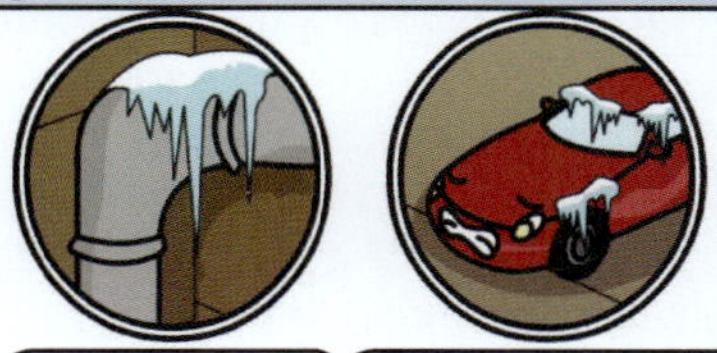

*"Pipe-Chilling"* **Piperacillin**

*"Tiny-Car-Chilling"* **Ticarcillin**

### Cephalosporins

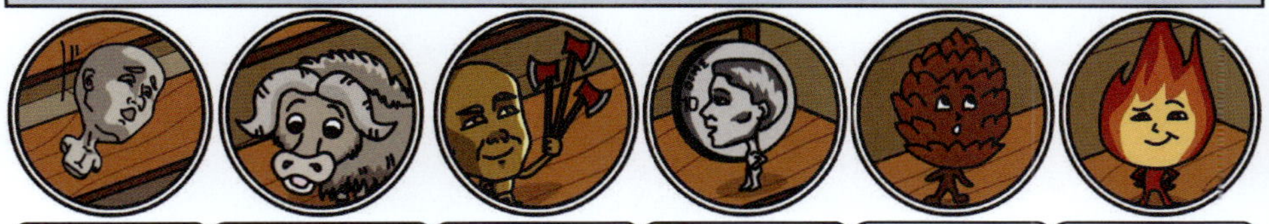

*"Ceph-Fall"* **Cephalexin**

*"Ceph-Furry-Ox"* **Cefuroxime**

*"Ceph-Tri-Axe"* **Ceftriaxone**

*"Ceph-Dime"* **Ceftazidime**

*"Ceph-Pine"* **Cefepime**

*"Ceph-Pyrc"* **Cefpirome**

### Others

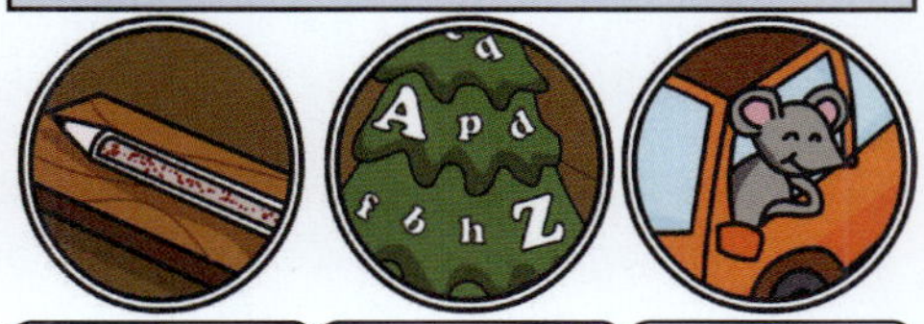

*"Marrow-Pen"* **Meropenem**

*"AZ-Tree"* **Aztreonam**

*"Van-Mice"* **Vancomycin**

☞ *"Ceph" stands for Cephalic, which is signified in the picture by the large heads of the Cephalosporins.*

# ANTIBACTERIAL DRUGS:
## INHIBIT NUCLEIC ACID SYNTHESIS

**Indications for antibacterial medications:** bacterial infections (UTIs, URTIs, LRTIs, sepsis, skin infections, etc), prophylaxis in patients with compromised immune systems.

**ANTIBIOTICS** act either by killing off bacteria directly or by inhibiting growth through altering cellular pathways involved in replication/reproduction. Various classes of antibiotics achieve this by inhibiting the synthesis of nucleic acids, examples include sulfonamides, dihydrofolate reductase inhibitors, quinolones, 5-nitroimidazoles, and DNA-dependant RNA polymerase inhibitors.

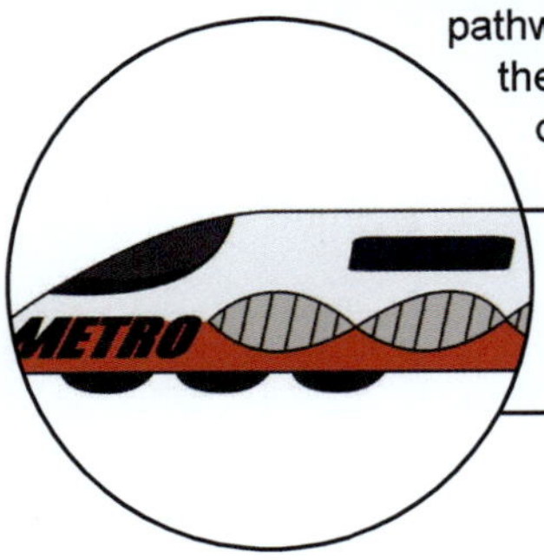


The DNA strand on the metro train remind you this picture is about antibiotics that inhibit nuclei acid synthesis.

### Sulphonamides

This class of antibiotics are made of a sulfonyl group connected to an amide group. This structure serves as a basic building block for different types of antibiotics with varying side chains. Sulfonamides hamper the growth of bacteria through competitively inhibiting an enzyme called dihydropteroate synthase (DHPS), which is needed for folate synthesis. Without adequate folate, bacteria are unable to divide and eventually bring its growth to a halt. ***Sulfadiazine***, ***sulfadoxine***, and ***sulfamethoxazole*** are examples of sulfonamide antibiotics. Sulfonamides are known for its potential to cause a fatal allergic reaction (type I hypersensitivity), but a more common allergic response these drugs are rashes and hives.

### Dihydrofolate Reductase Inhibitors

***Trimethoprim*** is an example of a commonly used dihydrofolate reductase inhibitor. Dihydrofolate reductase is an enzyme responsible for the reduction of dihydrofolic acid to tetrahydrofolic acid. This compound is needed for the synthesis of purine, thymidylic acid, and some amino acids needed for bacterial DNA synthesis. Trimethoprim is taken orally and is often used to treat bladder infection, middle ear infection, and traveler's diarrhea. Common side effects include nausea, vomiting or rash. In rare cases, it can suppress the bone marrow from producing white blood cells and lead to neutropenia.

### Quinolones

Quinolones are considered highly effective broad-spectrum antibiotics, and they cover both gram-positive and gram-negative bacteria. Examples of quinolones include ***levofloxacin***, ***norfloxacin***, ***ciprofloxacin***, and ***moxifloxacin***.

They are commonly used in genitourinary infections and to treat infections contracted in hospital either through direct contact or through invasive procedures like catheter insertion or surgeries.

Quinolones act by inhibiting DNA gyrase (topoisomerase II) and topoisomerase IV, which ultimately causes bacterial DNA to break into fragments and cause death to the cell. They are associated with tendonitis and tendon rupture as side effects, especially in patients who are on corticosteroids. Quinolones are contraindicated in patients who suffer from stroke, epilepsy or any central nervous system disorders.

### Nitroimidazoles

***Metronidazole*** is an antibacterial and antiprotozoal drug categorized under the drug class 5-nitroimidazoles. Metronidazole is an important drug for the treatment of colitis caused by Clostridium difficile. It is also effective against other protozoal infections such as vaginosis, endocarditis or pelvic inflammatory disease. Metronidazole inhibits nucleic acid synthesis through disruption of bacterial DNA, which subsequently prevents it from replicating. It is very common for patients who are on metronidazole to experience a "metallic" taste in the mouth and a whitened appearance of the tongue due to cell debris accumulation on the tongue papillae.

### RNA polymerase inhibitors

***Rifampicin***, also known as rifampin, is an example of a DNA-dependent RNA polymerase inhibitor. DNA-dependent RNA polymerase is an enzyme that is needed for DNA elongation and protein synthesis. This medication is commonly used for the treatment of bacterial infections, especially as part of tuberculosis treatment.

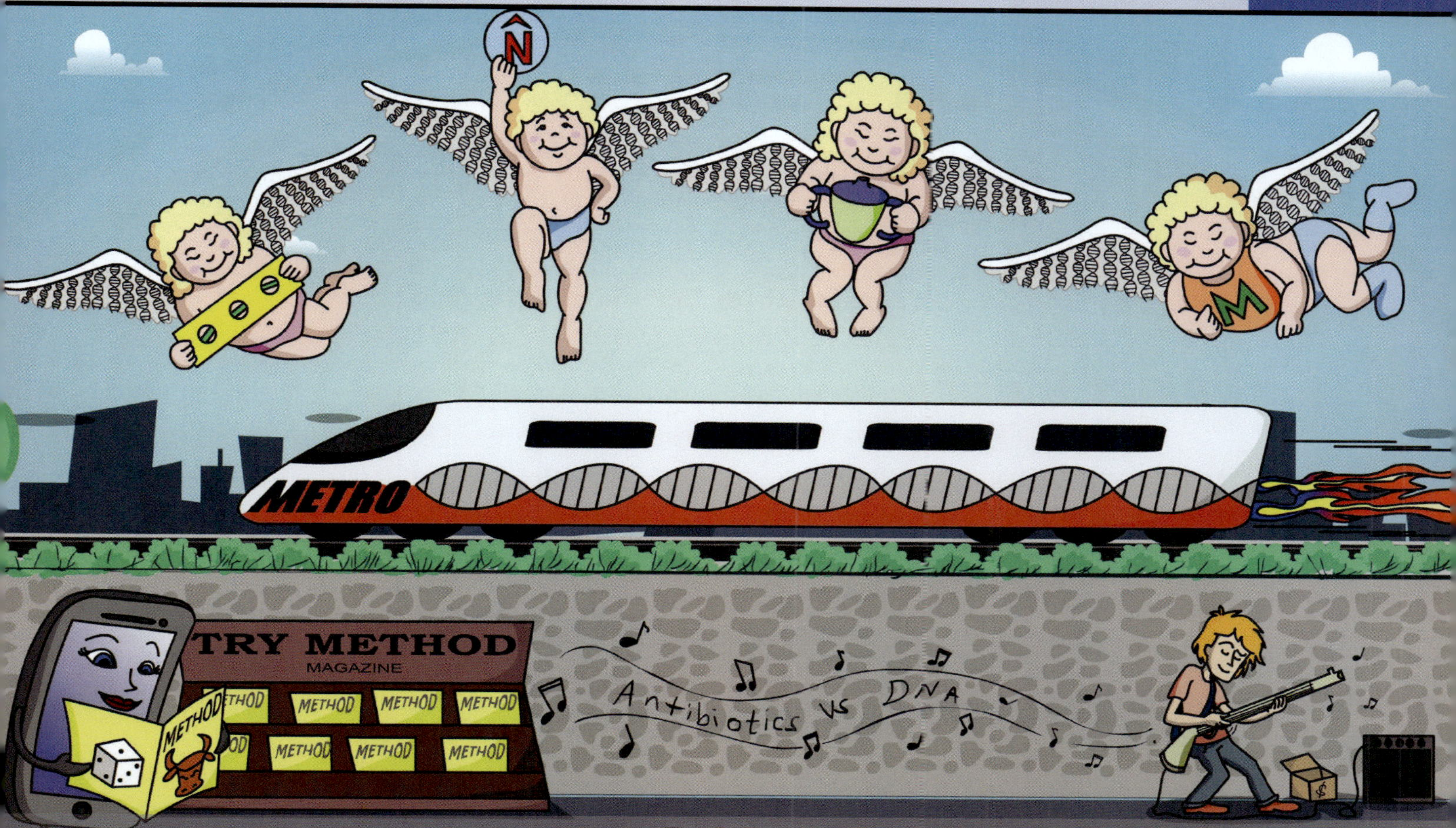


*The DNA train!*

## ANTIBACTERIAL DRUGS THAT INHIBIT NUCLEIC ACID SYNTHESIS

*The DNA strand on the metro train remind you this picture is about antibiotics thar inhibit nuclei acid synthesis.*

### Sulfonamides

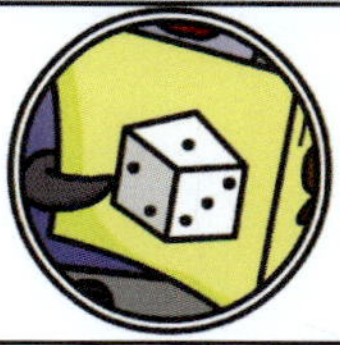

*"Cellphone-Die-Magazine"*
**Sulfadiazine**

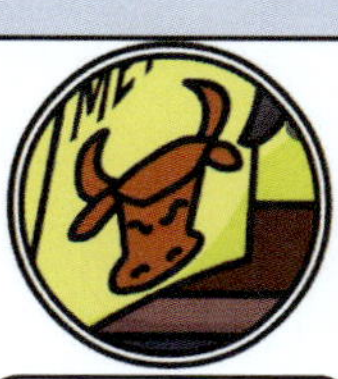

*"Cellphone-Ox"*
**Sulfadoxine**

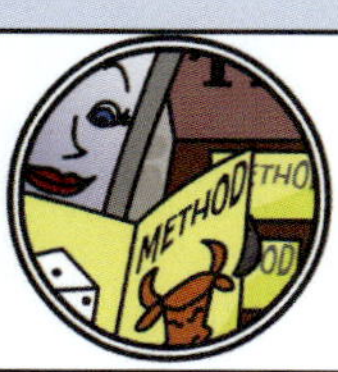

*"Cellphone-Method-Ox"*
**Sulfamethoxazole**

### Dihydrofolate Reductase inhibitors

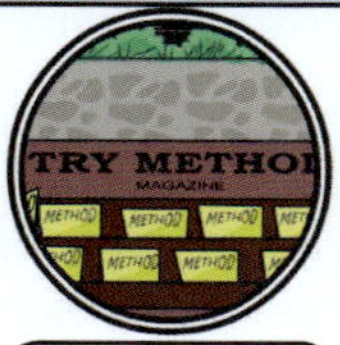

*"Try-Method"*
**Trimethoprim**

### Quinolones

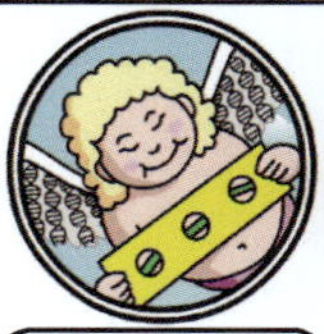

*"Level-Flock"*
**Levofloxacin**

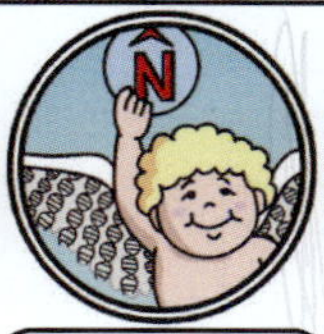

*"North-Flock"*
**Norfloxacin**

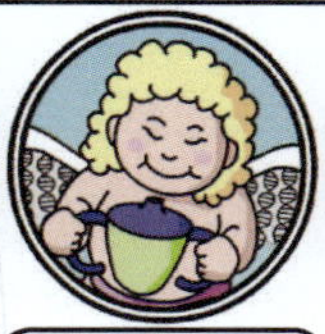

*"Sip-Flock"*
**Ciprofloxacin**

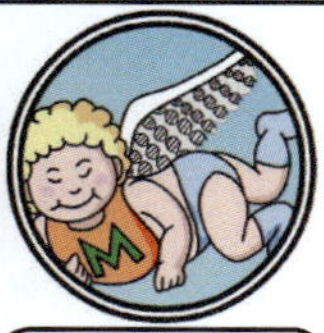

*"M-Flock"*
**Moxifloxacin**

*The quintuplets represent quinolones.*

### Nitroimidazoles

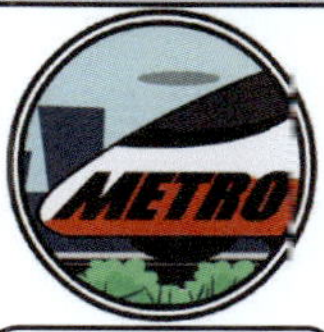

*"Metro"*
**Metronidazole**

### RNA polymerase inhibitor

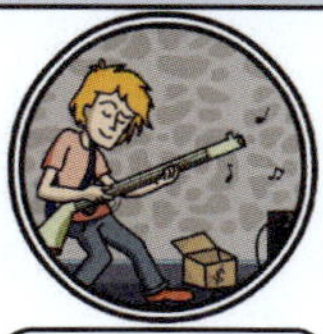

*"Rifle-Amp"*
**Rifampicin**

# ANTIBACTERIAL DRUGS:
## INHIBIT PROTEIN SYNTHESIS

**Indications for antibacterial medications:** bacterial infections (UTIs, URTIs, LRTIs, sepsis, skin infections, etc), prophylaxis in patients with compromised immune systems.

**ANTIBIOTICS INVOLVED IN PROTEIN SYNTHESIS INHIBITION** target the mRNA translation process. Therefore, hindrance of bacteria growth in this context takes place at the ribosomal level during the initiation, elongation, or termination phase of translation. Antibiotics that act through this mechanism are categorized as bacteriostatic agents and therefore must work together with the host immune system to ensure bacteria eradication.

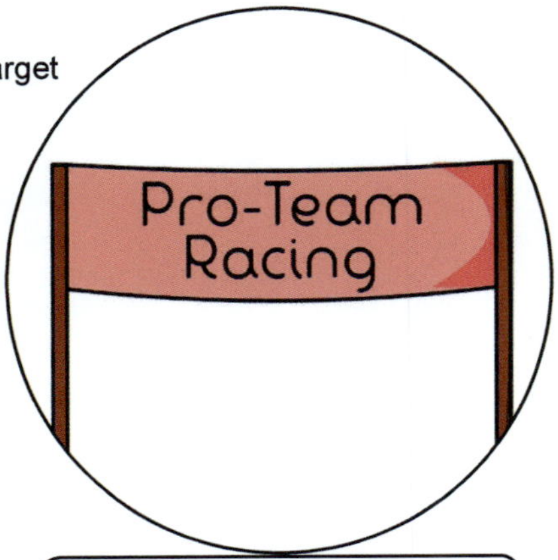


Pro-team (protein) racing reminds you this picture is about antibacterial drugs that inhibit protein synthesis.

### Macrolides

***Azithromycin***, ***clarithromycin***, and ***erythromycin***, are antibiotics that are capable of hindering bacterial growth by binding to the 50S ribosomal subunit and prevent translocation, leading to inhibition of polypeptide chain elongation. Macrolides are often used to treat strep throat caused by gram-positive Streptococcus species, and are often used in combination with other antibiotics to eradicate Helicobacter pylori infection.

### Aminoglycosides

***Neomycin***, ***gentamicin***, and ***amikacin*** bind to the 30S ribosomal subunit and lead to the incorrect reading of mRNA and the breakup of polysomes into monosomes. Ultimately, this causes protein synthesis and bacterial replication to fail. Aminoglycosides target gram-negative aerobes, and are used to treat severe infections of the abdomen, urinary tract, blood, and heart. Some aminoglycosides, like gentamicin, need to be monitored when administered due to risks of renal toxicity and ototoxicity.

### Tetracyclines

***Tetracycline, doxycycline, tigecycline,*** and ***minocycline*** bind to the 30S ribosomal subunits and block tRNA binding to the A site to the ribosome. They are often used to treat infections of the urinary, respiratory, and gastrointestinal tracts. Additionally, they can be used to treat moderate to severe acne, and in the treatment in chlamydia.

### Others

***Linezolid*** is an extremely important drug used against gram-positive bacteria that are resistant to other antibiotics. Its exact mechanism of action is not fully understood, but it may prevent protein synthesis through hindering mRNA from binding to the ribosomes before translation begins. Linezolid has a good safety profile and is often used in pregnant patients.

***Chloramphenicol*** acts by binding to the 50S ribosomal subunit and subsequently inhibiting the elongation phase of translation. It is used for the treatment of typhoid fever and acts as a second line agent for tetracycline resistant Cholera strains. One of the special features of Chloramphenicol is that it can penetrate the blood-brain barrier. Therefore, it is the drug of choice for the treatment of brain abscesses where the causative agent is unknown.

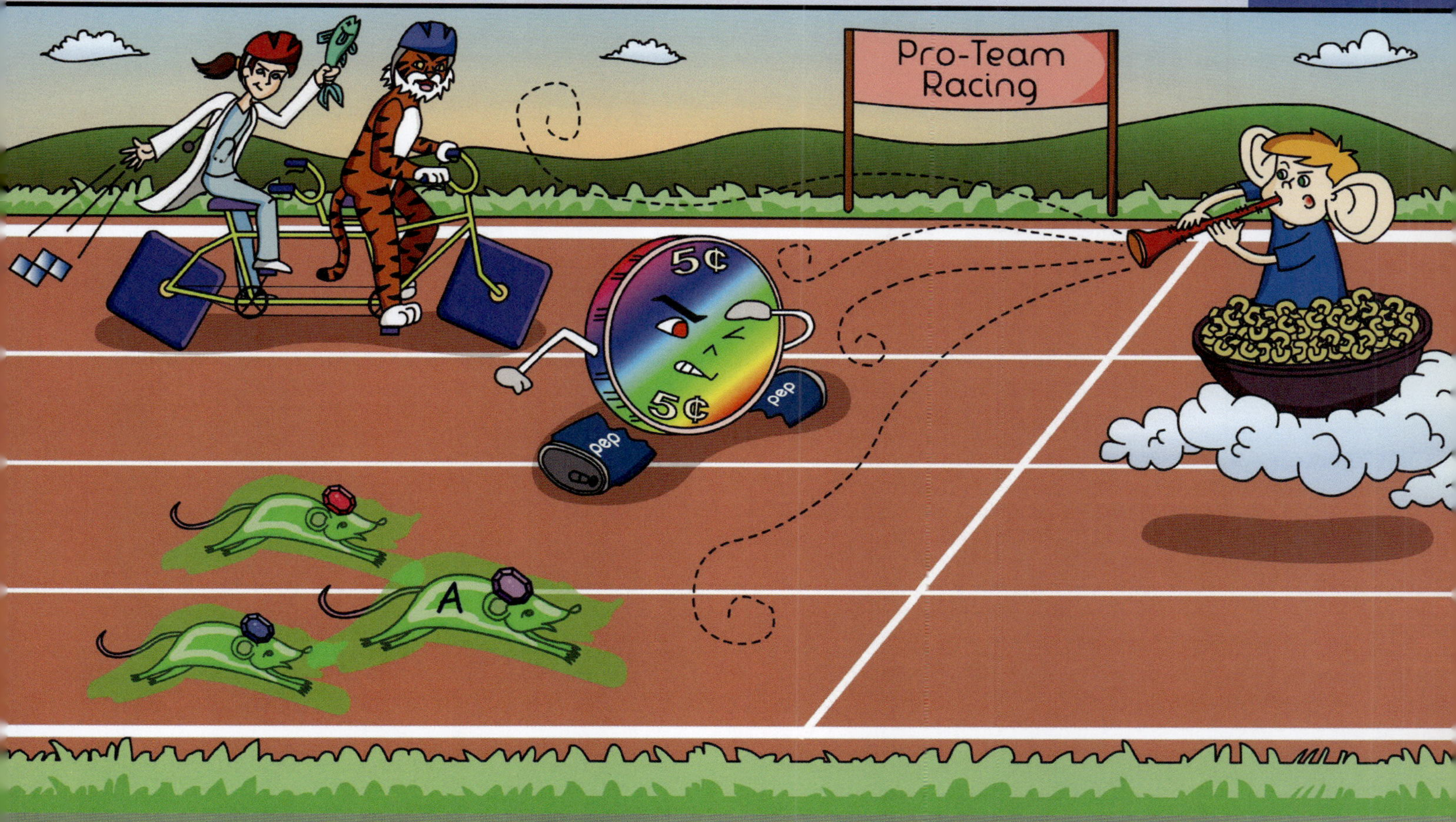


*Pro team racing!*

## ANTIBACTERIAL DRUGS THAT INHIBIT PROTEIN SYNTHESIS

☞ *Pro-team (protein) racing reminds you this picture is about antibacterial drugs that inhibit protein synthesis.*

### Macrolides 50

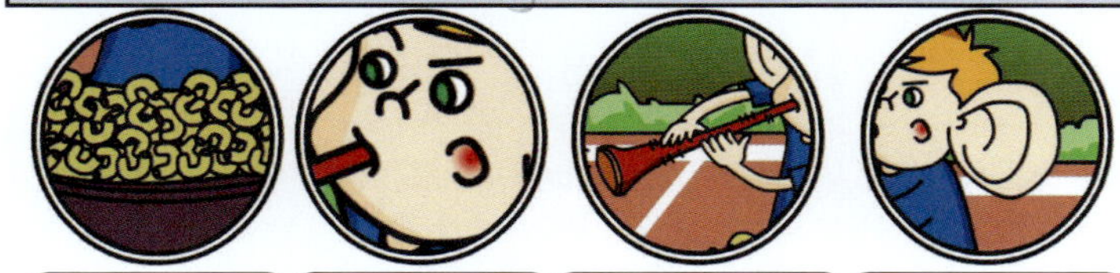

| "Macaroni" | "A-Zit" | "Clarinet" | "Ear" |
|---|---|---|---|
| Macrolides | Azithromycin | Clarithromycin | Erythromycin |

### Aminoglycosides 30

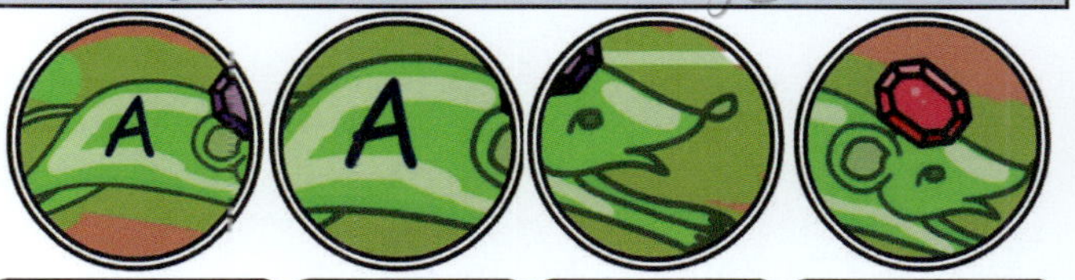

| "A" | "A-Mice" | "Neon-Mice" | "Gem-Mice" |
|---|---|---|---|
| Aminoglycosides | Amikacin | Neomycin | Gentamicin |

### Tetracyclines 30 (tRNA)

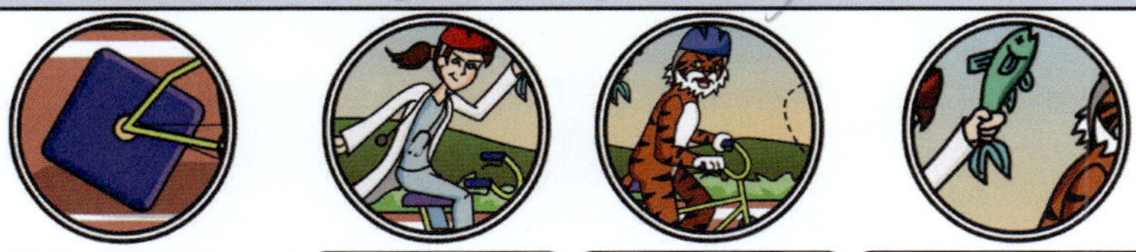

| "Tetra[four]-Cycling" | "Doc-Cycling" | "Tiger-Cycling" | "Minnow-Cycling" |
|---|---|---|---|
| Tetracycline | Doxycycline | Tigecycline | Minocycline |

### Other

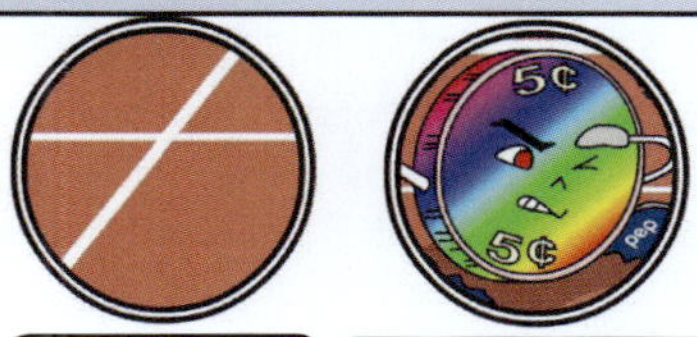

50

| "Lines" | "Colorful-Nickel" |
|---|---|
| Linezolid | Chloramphenicol |

# ANTIVIRALS

**Indications for antiviral medications:** viral infections (HSV, CMV, herpes, hepatitis B, influenza A & B, HIV, HBV, etc.), is also used as prophylaxis in some instances.

**ANTIVIRAL DRUGS** are used to combat viral infections. Mechanisms of action include DNA polymerase inhibitors, reverse transcriptase inhibitors (RTIs), protease inhibitors, HIV entry inhibitors, uncoating inhibitors, neuraminidase inhibitors, and immunomodulators.

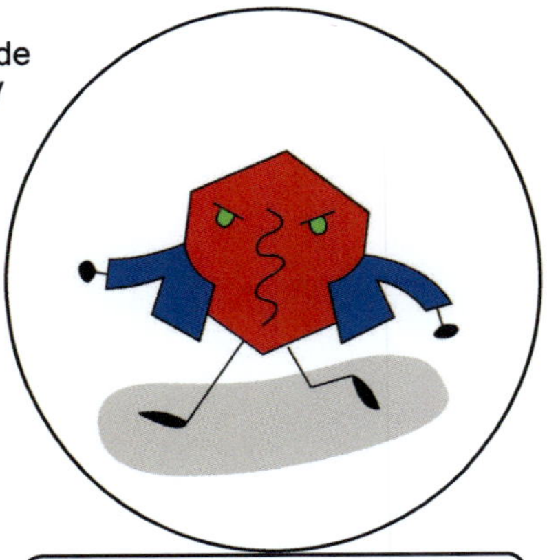

The red characters represent viruses invading the cell (castle), and will remind you this picture is about antivirals.

## DNA Polymerase Inhibitors

DNA polymerase inhibitors, such as ***acyclovir***, ***famciclovir***, and ***ganciclovir*** competitively bind to viral DNA polymerase and prevent it from synthesizing DNA. These medications are commonly used for the treatment of infections caused by herpes simplex virus (HSV), epstein barr virus (EBV) and varicella zoster virus (VZV or chicken pox). Intravenous administration of acyclovir should be monitored carefully as it can lead to nephrotoxicity due to the accumulation of acyclovir crystals in the kidney.

## Reverse Transcriptase Inhibitors (RTIs): NRTI and NNRTI

Some viruses, such as human immunodeficiency virus (HIV), require reverse transcriptase for the synthesis of complementary DNA from their RNA template. A class of antiviral drugs known as the reverse transcriptase inhibitors (RTI) targets this process. RTIs are classified into either nucleoside (NRTI) and non-nucleoside (NNRTI) subtypes based on their chemical structures. Examples of NRTIs include ***lamivudine*** and ***zidovudine***, and examples of NNRTIs include ***efavirenz*** and ***nevirapine***.

A combination therapy referred to as the highly active antiretroviral therapy (HAART) treatment regime use a number of RTIs to treat HIV or AIDS, and although it can't cure the disease, it can prevent it from being fatal. NRTIs and NNRTIs act by inhibiting reverse transcriptase and preventing synthesis of DNA from viral RNA. Common side effects include nausea, vomiting, heartburn, headache, and in rare cases, might lead to white blood cell deficiency and liver toxicity.

## Protease Inhibitors

The next class of antiviral drugs are the protease inhibitors. Unlike NRTIs, the protease inhibitors prevent viral spread through binding to protease enzymes, making them unable to cleave post-translational proteins into infectious viral particles. This class of drug is often used as part of the HIV combination therapy, and to treat the hepatitis C virus. Some examples of protease inhibitors are ***saquinavir***, ***atazanavir*** and ***ritonavir***. Protease inhibitors are associated with side effects such as hyperlipidemia and kidney stones.

## HIV entry Inhibitors

***Enfuvirtide*** is an antiviral drug that inhibits the entry of viruses into host cells. It is effective in combating HIV-1 through changing the chemical configuration of viral antigen and therefore preventing it from fusing with target host cells. Enfuvirtide is mainly administered intravenously, so it can lead to pain and redness at the site of injection. In some cases, it can cause tingling sensation at the extremities, loss of appetite, and joint pain.

## Uncoating Inhibitors

***Amantadine*** is an antiviral drug that blocks M2 protein channels on the virus. This mechanism disrupts the viral uncoating process in the host cells and prevents viral RNA transcription. It is mainly used for the treatment of Influenza virus infections. Amantadine is also capable of blocking NMDA-type glutamate receptors and preventing dopamine reuptake, allowing this medication to be beneficial in the treatment of Parkinson's disease.

## Neuraminidase Inhibitors

Neuraminidase is a viral enzyme that facilitates viral particles exiting the host cell and infecting new cells. ***Oseltamivir*** and ***zanamivir*** inhibit this enzyme to prevent exit of the virus from the cell.

## Immunomodulators

***Interferon-alpha*** is a protein that regulates host's immune system. It acts by binding to the interferon receptors and sending signals to the host immune cells to attack the viruses.

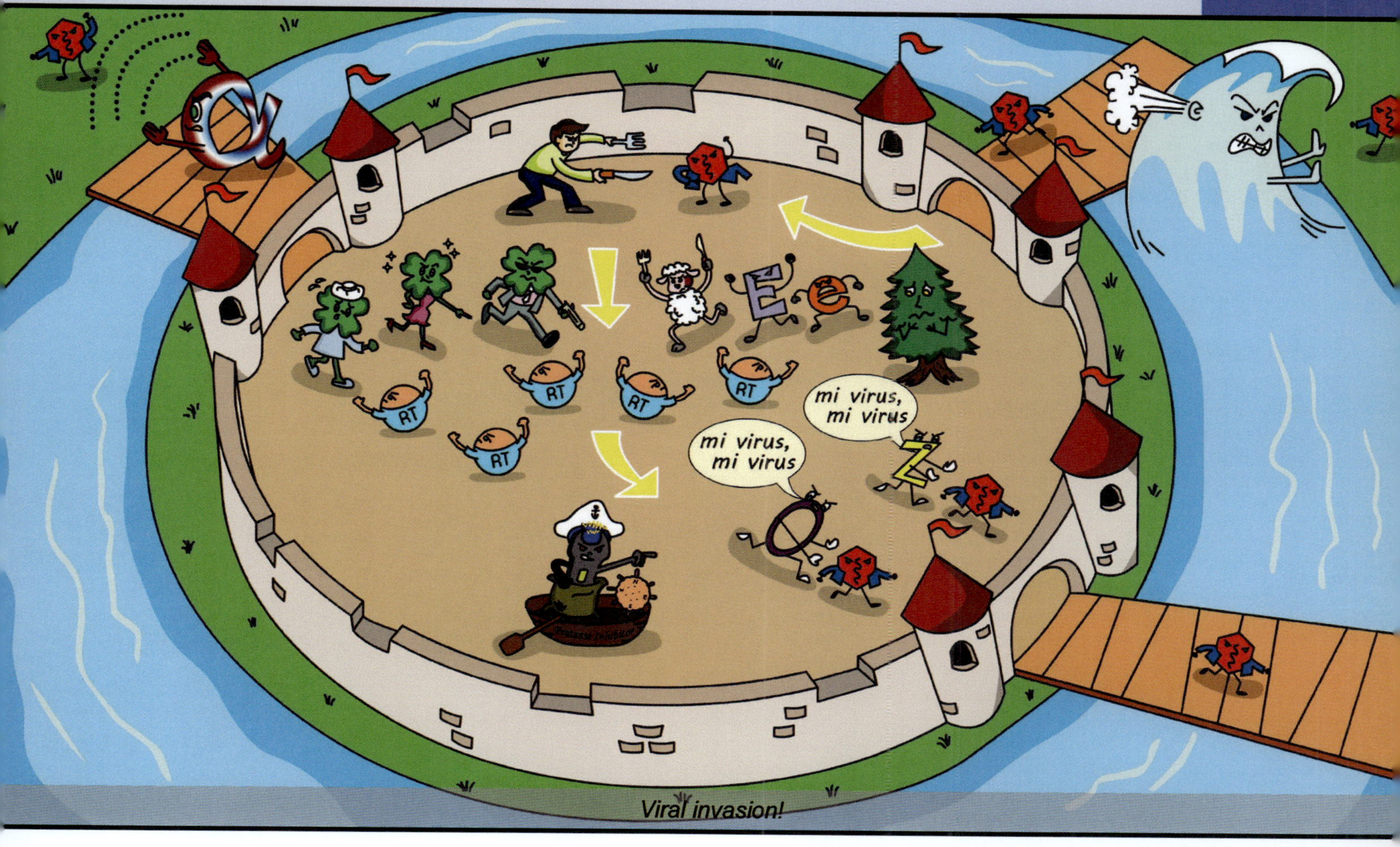


## ANTIVIRALS

*The red characters represent viruses invading the cell (castle), and will remind you this picture is about antivirals.*

### DNA Polymerase Inhibitors

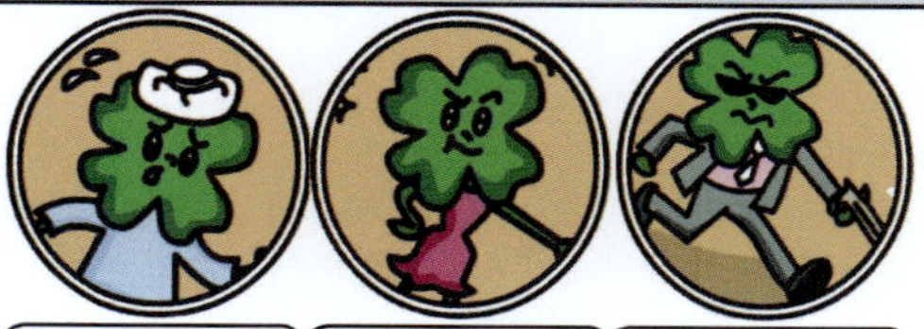

"A-Sick-Clover" **Acyclovir**

"Famous-Clover" **Famciclovir**

"Gangster-Clover" **Ganciclovir**

### NRTI

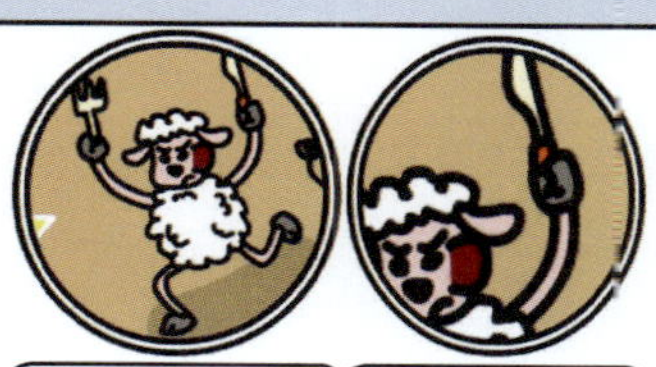

"Lamb-Dine" **Lamivudine**

"Zit-Dine" **Zidovudine**

### NNRTI

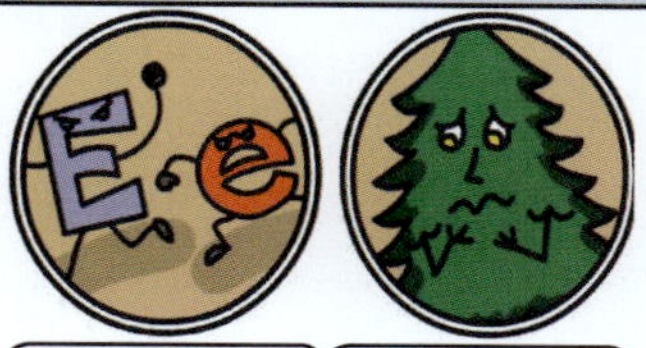

"E-Friends" **Efavirenz**

"Nervous-Pine" **Nevirapine**

### Protease Inhibitors

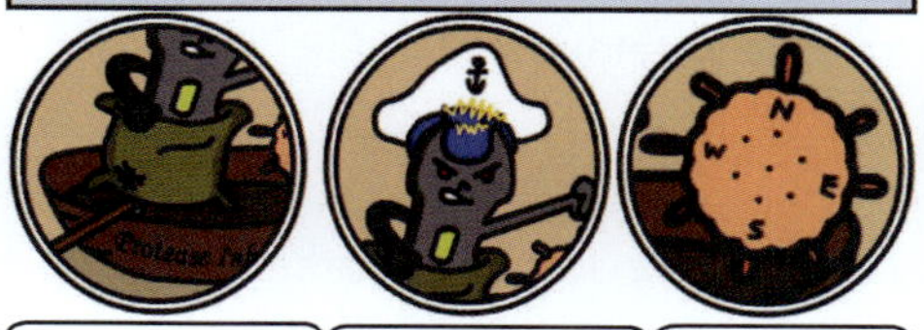

"Sack-Navigator" **Saquinavir**

"A-Tazor-Navigator" **Atazanavir**

"Ritz-Navigator" **Ritonavir**

### Inhibit HIV entry

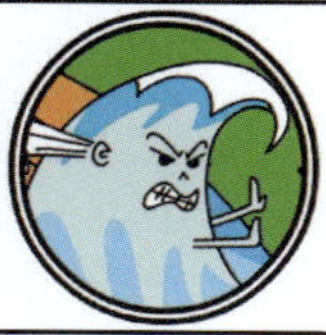

"Furious-Tide" **Enfuvirtide**

### Inhibit Uncoating

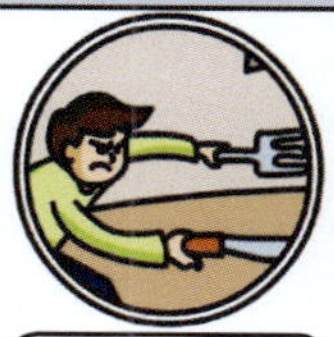

"A-Man-Dine" **Amantadine**

### Inhibit Exit

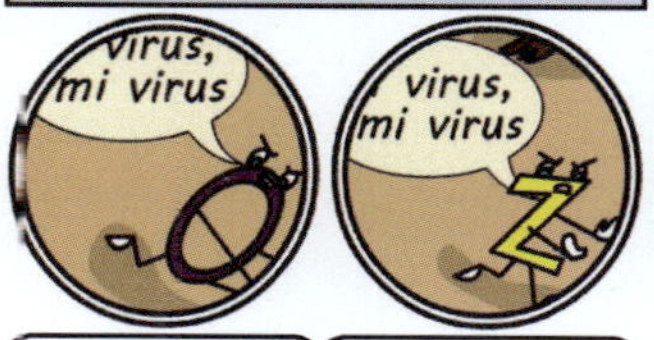


"O-Mi-Virus" **Oseltamivir**

"Z-Mi-Virus" **Zanamivir**

### Immunomodulators

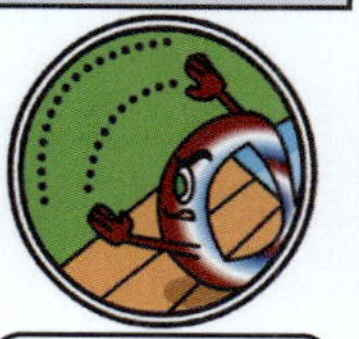

"Interfere-Alpha" **Interferon-Alpha**

# ANTIHELMINTICS

**Indications for antihelmintic medications:** helminth infections (roundworms, flatworms, flukes, tapeworms).

**HELMINTH INFECTIONS** are described as the infestation of parasitic worms into host body tissues. The parasites do not typically kill their host, but instead, live inside their bodies while receiving nutrition and protection. Over long periods of time, this may cause the host to become nutritionally deficient and render them prone to other infections. Most helminthes do not multiply or proliferate, but the disease state depends on a number of factors such as the parasite load, host immune system, and concomitant presence of other infections.

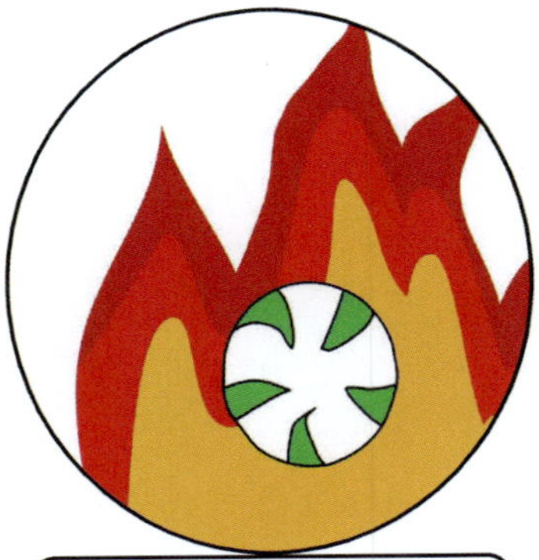

The "hell-mints" remind you this picture is about antihelmintics!

Parasites can be classified into four categories: nematodes (roundworms), platyhelminthes (flatworms), trematodes (flukes) and cestodes (tapeworms). They invade into the host either through oral ingestion, arthropod bites, or penetration of skin.

## Intestinal Nematodes

The anthelmintic drugs effective against intestinal nematodes include ***mebendazole***, ***albendazole***, and ***piperazine***.

***Mebendazole*** may be used alone to treat mild to moderate helminth infestation. It acts by inhibiting the synthesis of microtubules and prevents the parasite's ability to absorb nutrients from the host intestinal cells. This drug is taken orally in the form of a capsule and has relatively slow onset of action. In more severe cases, the use of mebendazole alone may cause the parasites to migrate out of the intestines leading to complications such as acute appendicitis, intestinal perforation, or peritonitis. It is therefore recommended to be used with ***piperazine*** which paralyzes the parasites and prevents them from migrating to other sites and, as a result, the parasites are excreted in the feces of the host.

## Tissue Nematodes

Tissue nematodes such as filaria can be treated with ***ivermectin*** and ***diethylcarbamazine***.

***Ivermectin*** acts by binding to glutamate gated chloride channels located in the membrane of muscle and nerve cells. This increases the membrane's permeability to chloride ions and leads to hyperpolarization. The end result is an inhibitory effect to neurotransmission in parasites. Ivermectin has a wide spectrum of indications as it can also be used to treat lice infection, scabies, and strongyloidiasis. This drug can be taken orally or it can be applied as a topical cream and in severe cases can be administered intravenously for a more rapid effect. The side effect of ivermectin is neurotoxicity which leads to disorders in coordination of body movement or CNS depression.

Unlike ivermectin, ***diethylcarbamazine*** inhibits the metabolism of arachidonic acid in microfilariae, thereby inducing the host immune system to attack the parasite instead of killing it directly.

## Platyhelminths: Trematodes (Flukes)

Trematodes are parasitic flatworms classified under the phylum platyhelminthes and are commonly known as flukes. This parasite can cause infectious diseases such as schistosomiasis, and can be treated effectively with the use of ***praziquantel***.

Although praziquantel's exact mechanism of action is not well understood, it is thought that it is able to alter the permeability of the cell membrane and increase calcium ion influx. As a result, the parasite becomes strongly contracted and eventually dies secondary to paralysis. Similar to other anthelmintic drugs, praziquantel is usually taken orally. Common side effects of include abdominal pain, nausea, headache, and allergic reaction.

## Platyhelminths: Cestodes (Tapeworms)

Cestodes, also called tapeworms, can be eliminated from the host body using ***praziquantel*** and ***niclosamide***.

***Niclosamide*** acts by inhibiting cellular respiration through blocking glucose uptake and oxidative phosphorylation, processes which are vital for the survival of the parasite. Niclosamide is not effective against treating other parasites such as pinworms or roundworms. Common side effects include nausea, vomiting, constipation, drowsiness, skin rash, and perianal itching.

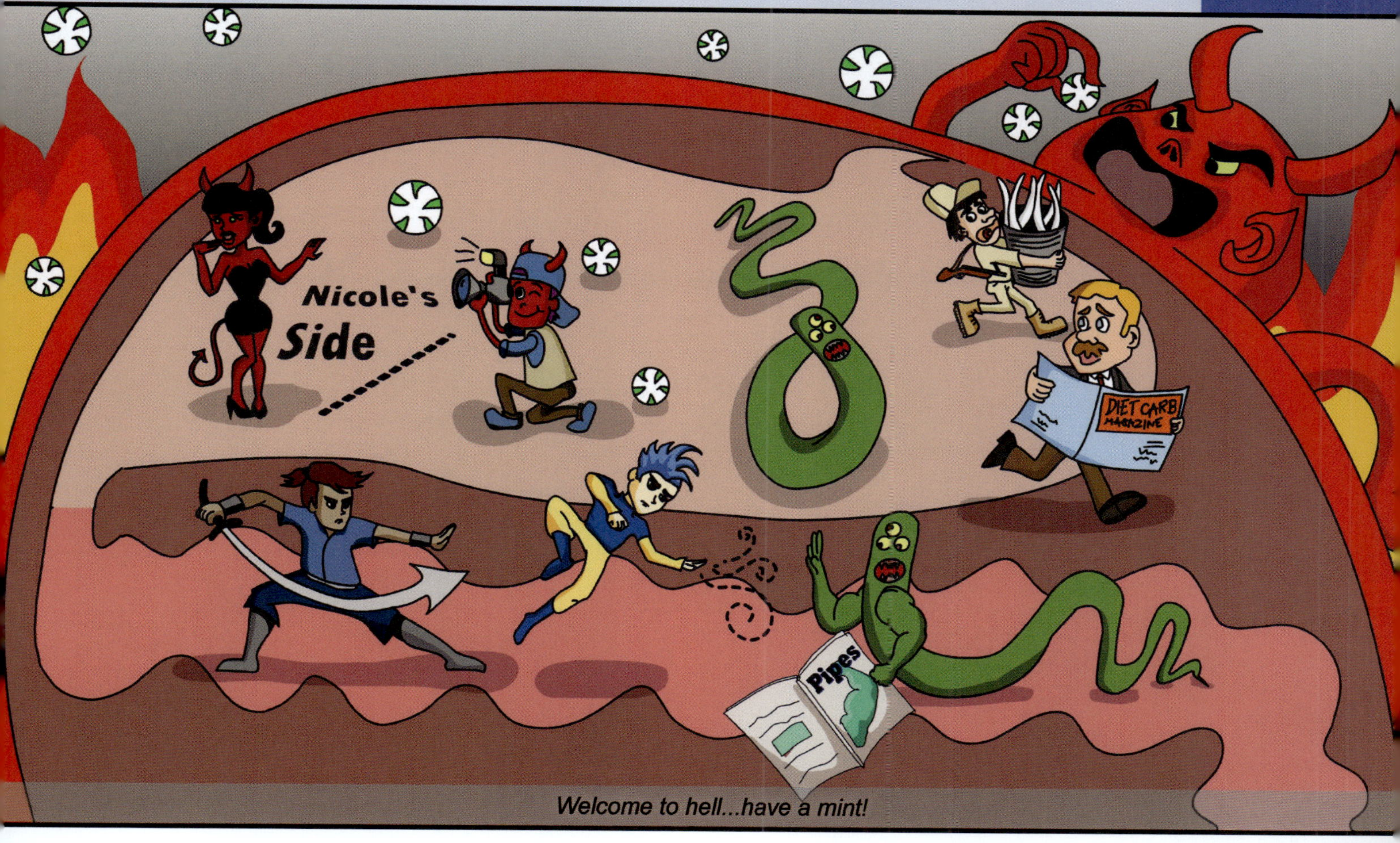


## ANTIHELMINTICS

The "*hell-mints*" remind you this picture is about anti*helmint*ics!

### Intestinal Nematodes

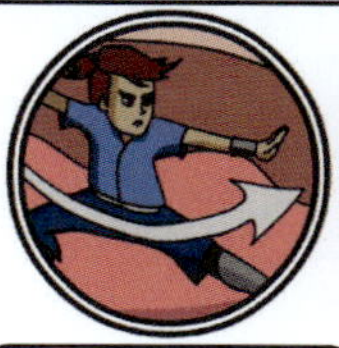

"Metal-Bender"
**Mebendazole**

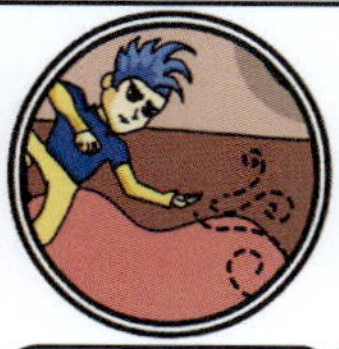

"Air-Bender"
**Albendazole**

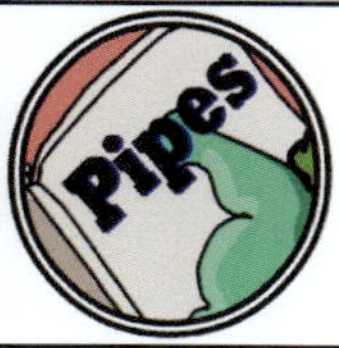


"Pipe-Magazine"
**Piperazine**

### Tissue Nematodes

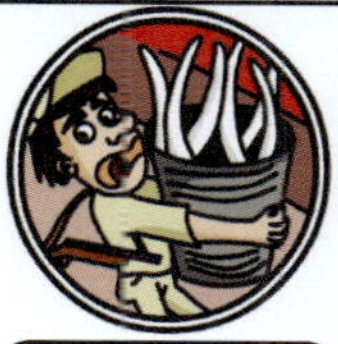

"Ivory-Tin"
**Ivermectin**

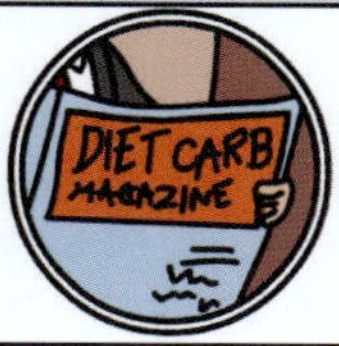


"Diet-Carb-Magazine"
**Diethylcarbamazine**

### Platyhelminths: Trematodes

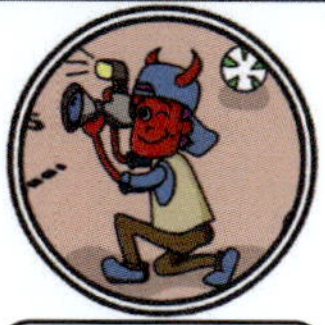

"Paparazzi"
**Praziquantel**

### Platyhelminths: Cestodes

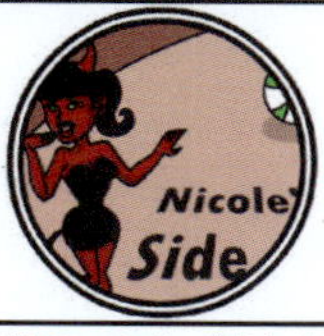


"Nicole's-Side"
**Niclosamide**

# ANTIFUNGALS

**Indications for antifungal medications:** fungal infections (tinea pedis, tinea cruris, tinea corporis, candida, invasive candidiasis, etc).

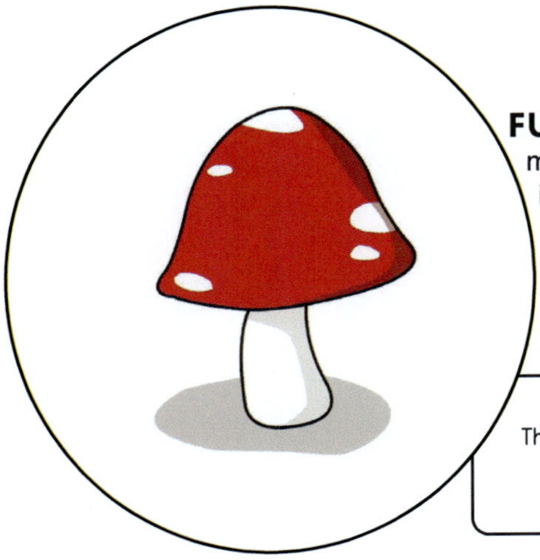

**FUNGAL INFECTIONS** are infections caused by spore-forming microorganisms such as yeast and moulds. Generally, people who are immunocompromised; such as patients on chemotherapy, patients with HIV infection, or those who are on corticosteroid treatment; are at a higher risk of contracting fungal infections.

The mushrooms (fungus) reminds you of antifungals!

## Polyenes

Polyenes, such as ***amphotericin***, are a group of antifungal drugs that target cholesterol molecules called ergosterol found on the surface of fungal cell membranes. The osmotic pressure difference between the inside and outside of the cell membrane causes leakage of sodium and potassium ions, and as a result, regulation of homeostasis is disrupted and fungal cell death occurs. These drugs are effective against yeast infections in genital organs and oral thrush.

## Azoles

Azole antifungal drugs act by binding to phospholipids in the fungal cell membrane and inhibit the biosynthesis of ergosterol and other sterols required for cell membrane integrity. Azoles can be subgrouped into imidazoles and triazoles. The two subgroups only differ from each other in their molecular structure. ***Ketoconazole***, ***miconazole,*** and ***clotrimazole*** are examples of imidazoles, while ***fluconazole***, ***itraconazole,*** and ***voriconazole*** are part of the triazole subgroup.

## Echinocandins

Echinocandins, such as ***caspofungin***, act by binding onto the surface of an enzyme called 1,3-beta glucan synthase, and inhibiting the formation of cell walls made of glucan. The echinocandins exhibit both fungicidal and fungistatic properties, depending on the type of fungi. This group of drugs are associated with increase in liver enzymes.

## Allylamines

Allylamines are a class of antifungals effective for the treatment of dermatophytosis, such as athlete's foot and onychomycosis. These drugs come in the form of topical ointments or they can be taken orally. ***Terbinafine*** is an example of an allylamine. Its mechanism of action is through disrupting fungal cell membrane synthesis through inhibition of sterol production.

## Others

***Flucytosine*** is often used in combination with polyenes to manage more severe fungal infections as flucytosine alone is not effective against killing fungi, but can be used to potentiate and synergize the fungicidal properties of other antifungal drugs. Flucytosine is usually used in combination with amphotericin B or azole antifungals and, as it is unclear to whether it affects fetal growth, should be avoided in pregnant women.

***Griseofulvin*** is an antifungal drug used for the treatment of dermatophytosis if other first line agents are ineffective. It acts by inhibiting mitosis through binding to tubulin.

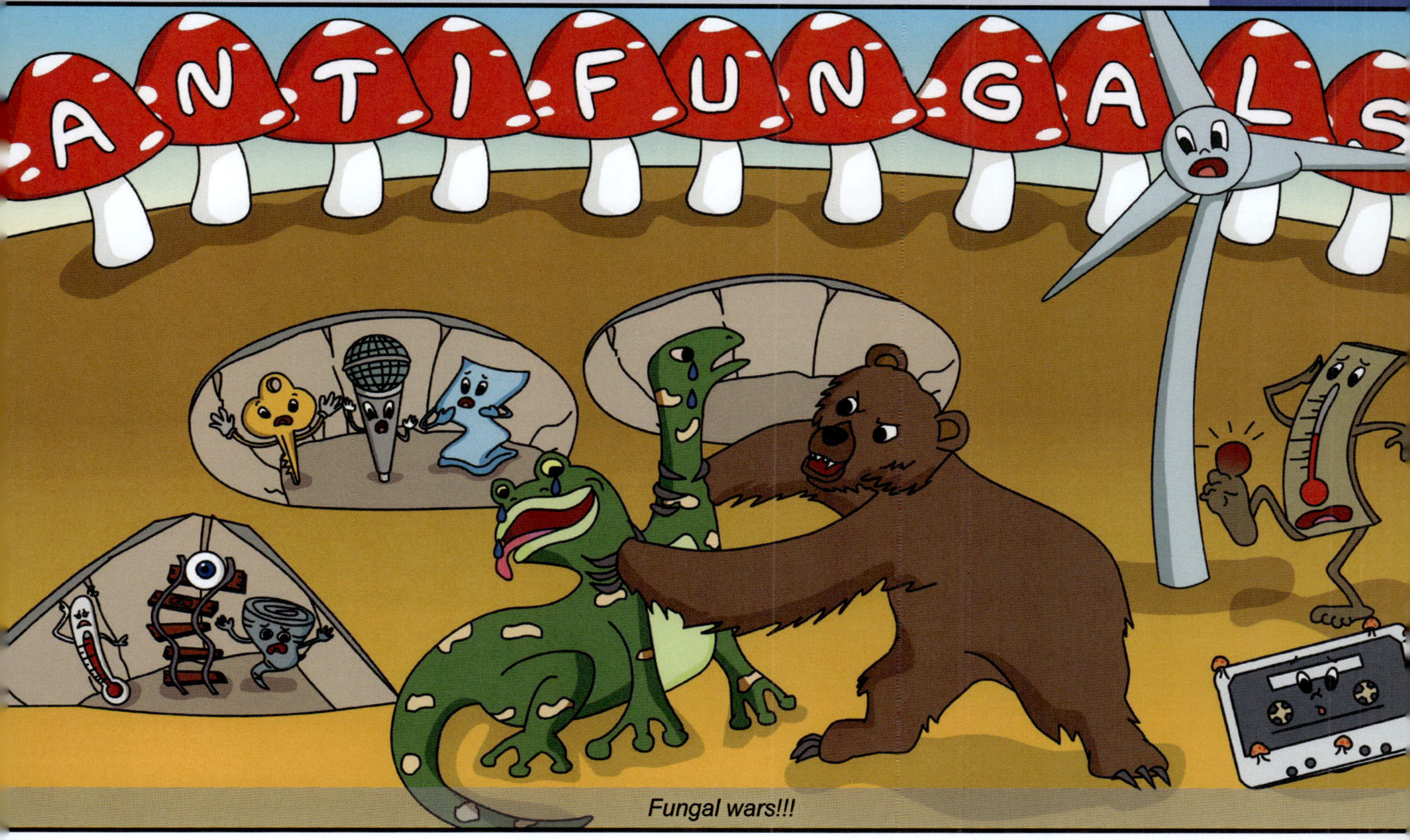

Fungal wars!!!

## ANTIFUNGALS

*The mushrooms (fungus) reminds you of antifungals!*

### Polyenes

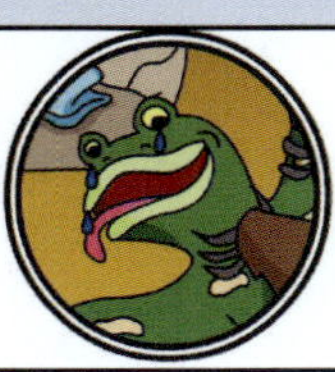

*"Amphibian-Tears"*
**Amphotericin**

### Azoles: Imidazoles

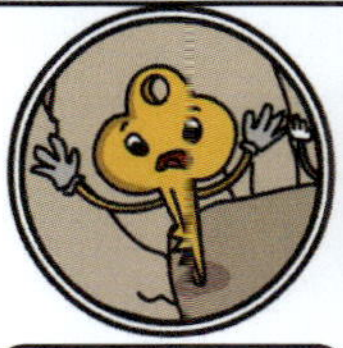

*"Key-A-Hole"*
**Ketoconazole**

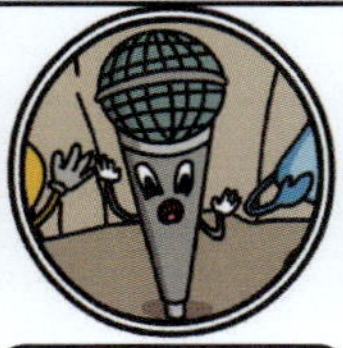

*"Mic-A-Hole"*
**Miconazole**

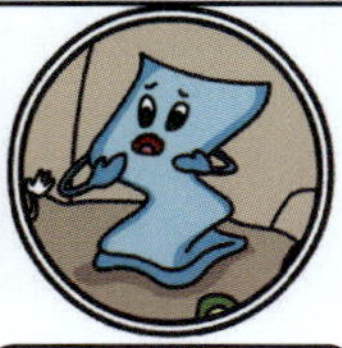

*"Cloth-A-Hole"*
**Clotrimazole**

### Azoles: Triazoles

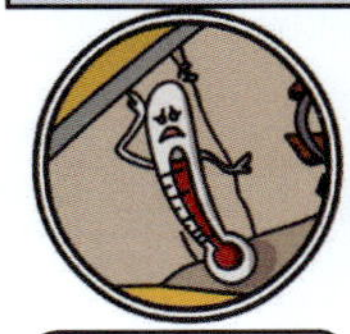

*"Flu-A-Hole"*
**Fluconazole**

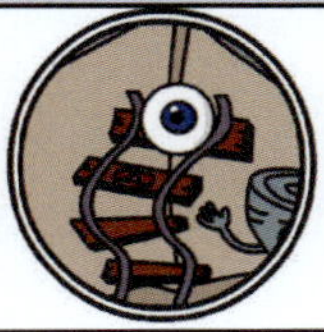

*"Eye-Track-A-Hole"*
**Itraconazole**

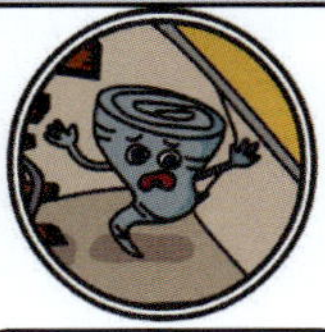

*"Vortex-A-Hole"*
**Voriconazole**

### Echinocandins

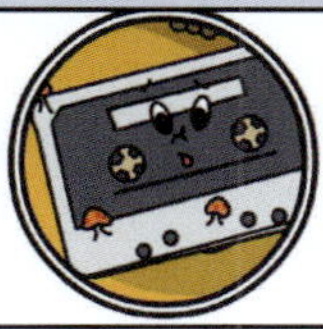

*"Casette-Fungus"*
**Caspofungin**

### Allylamines

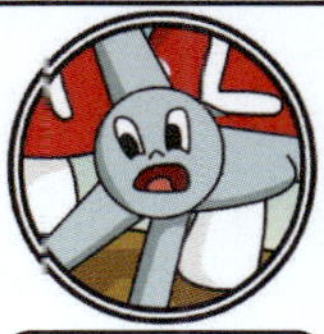

*"Terbine"*
**Terbinafine**

### Others

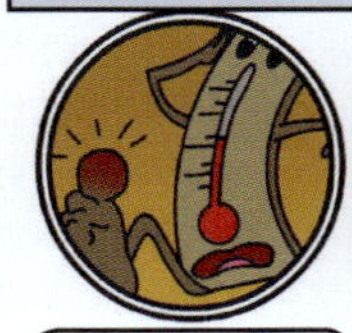

*"Flu-Toe"*
**Flucytosine**

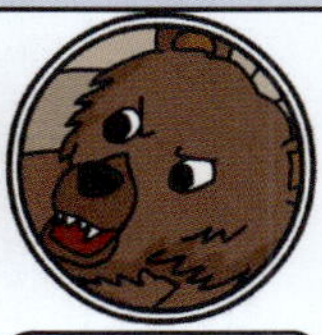

*"Grizzily"*
**Griseofulvin**

*The three-sided hole contains the triazoles, and the middle-hole contains the imidazoles.*

# ANTIMALARIALS

**Indications for antimalarials:** malaria prophylaxis and treatment.

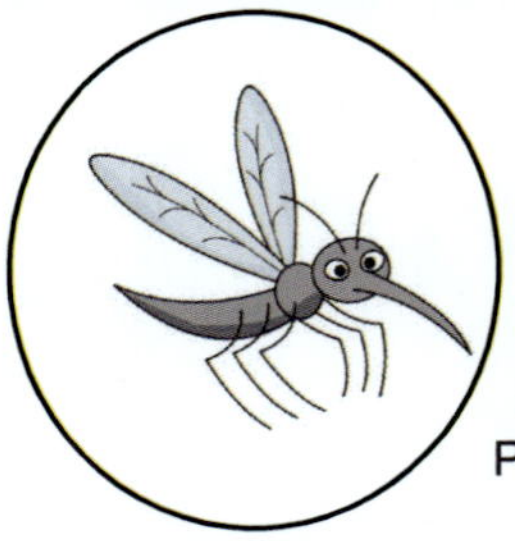

**MALARIA** is a serious infectious disease commonly transmitted by infected female Anopheles mosquitoes. It can also be passed on from mother to child through blood transfusion or through sharing needles. The disease is caused by parasitic protozoans of the Plasmodium type. There are five species of Plasmodium that can infect humans: Plasmodium falciparum, Plasmodium vivax, Plasmodium ovale, Plasmodium malariae, and Plasmodium knowlesi.

The mosquitoes remind you this picture is about malaria.

The cardinal symptoms of malaria are malaise, fever, muscle aches, anorexia, and rigor. Patients might also present with signs such as anemia, thrombocytopenia, jaundice, hepatosplenomegaly, and renal dysfunction. The goal of treatment is to eliminate the parasite from the body and to prevent the occurrence of complications.

## Tissue Schizonticides

Tissue schizonticides, for example ***primaquine***, primarily act on Plasmodium that reside and grow in liver tissues. By blocking the growth of parasites, the development of infection can be prevented.

Primaquine is generally used for prophylactic purposes, specifically to prevent the relapse of malaria caused by P. vivax and P. ovale. The common side effects of primaquine include nausea, vomiting, and abdominal cramps. It must be noted that primaquine should not be taken by people who have glucose-6-phosphate deficiency (G6PD) as the drug may lead to lysis of red blood cells followed by severe systemic complications.

## Blood Schizonticides

Blood schizonticides eliminate plasmodia from the body by targeting red blood cells in which the parasite has invaded. These drugs can be classified based on their duration of action: slow or fast acting. ***Proguanil*** and ***pyrimethamine*** are considered slow-acting, while ***quinine***, ***mefloquine***, and ***chloroquine*** are fast-acting.

## Slow Acting

***Proguanil*** acts through its active metabolite, cycloguanil, that is able to inhibit dihydrofolate reductase, an enzyme responsible for folic acid synthesis in the parasite. Its inhibition prevents the parasite from forming DNA and amino acids required for parasitic growth. The drug is usually taken orally in combination with chloroquine and side effects include skin rashes, abdominal discomfort, diarrhea, and skin itchiness. The drug is metabolized in the liver and kidney, so patients who have functional impairment of these organs should avoid taking proguanil to prevent drug accumulation in circulation.

***Pyrimethamine*** is primarily active against P. falciparum and P. vivax. Due to the increase in pyrimethamine resistant parasites, there has been a decreased use of this drug and is now typically used only in conjunction with other malaria medications.

## Fast Acting

***Quinine*** is effective against P. falciparum. This drug is able to disrupt the ability of the malaria parasite to metabolize hemoglobin for its own trophic purposes. This leads to the accumulation of cytotoxic heme in the red blood cells and the eventual death of the parasites. Side effects include tinnitus, sweating, and rarely may cause deafness, thrombocytopenia, and cardiac arrhythmia.

***Mefloquine*** is often used as prevention for malarial infections. It is taken one to two weeks before exposure and treatment continues until exposure is discontinued. It can also be used to treat infections, particularly with chloroquine resistant P. falciparum and P. vivax.

***Chloroquine***'s exact mechanism of action is unknown. It is effective in treating and preventing infections against P. vivax, P. ovale, and P. malariae, however, is less effective in treating infections caused by P. falciparum due to drug resistance. The most commonly reported side effects include muscle ache, skin rashes, and diarrhea. In more severe cases, the drug can lead to cytopenia, seizures, and vision disturbances.

## Antibiotics and Other Antimalarials

***Artemether*** and ***lumefantrine***'s mechanism of action is unknown. These two medications are often used in combination to treat malaria caused by P. falciparum that is not responsive to chloroquine. It should be noted that this drug is associated with hypersensitivity reactions and can lead to anaphylaxis.

Antibiotics, such as ***doxycycline*** and ***sulfadoxine***, are also used to treat and prevent malaria in combination with first line antimalarial drugs.

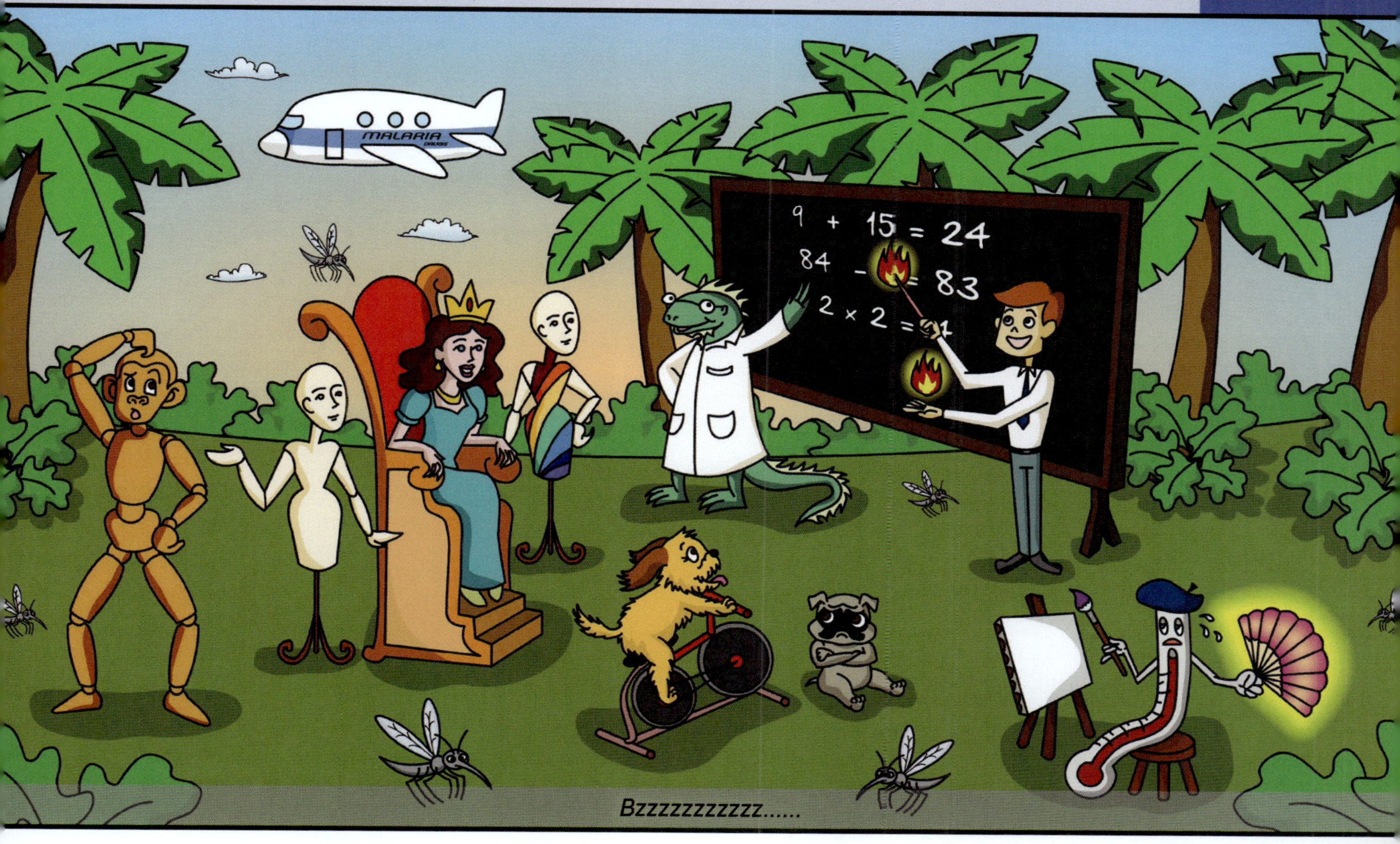


## ANTIMALARIALS

*The mosquitoes remind you this picture is about malaria!*

### Tissue Schizonticide

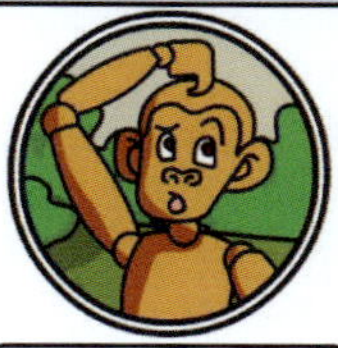

*"Primate-Mannequin"*
**Primaquine**

### Blood Schizonticide: Slow

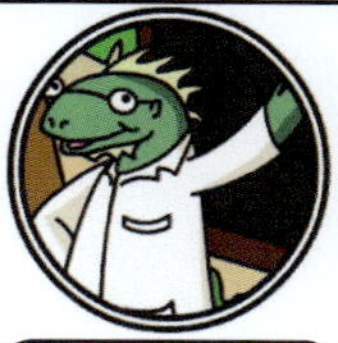

*"Prof-Iguana"*
**Proguanil**

*"Pyro-Math-Man"*
**Pyrimethamine**

### Blood Schizonticide: Fast

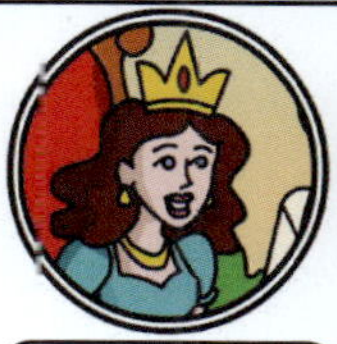

*"Queen"*
**Quinine**

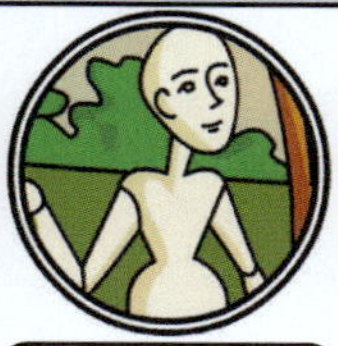

*"Mannequin"*
**Mefloquine**

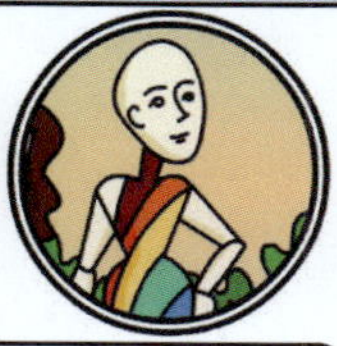

*"Color-Mannequin"*
**Chloroquine**

### Others

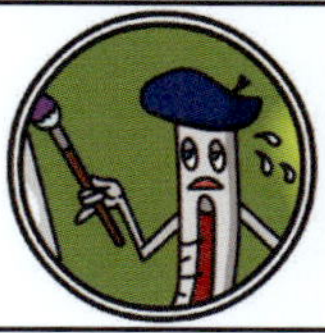

*"Art-Thermometer"*
**Artemether**

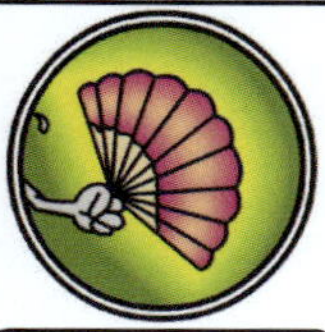

*"Luminous-Fan"*
**Lumefantrine**

### Antibiotics

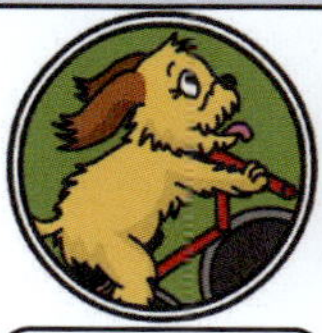

*"Dog-Cycling"*
**Doxycycline**

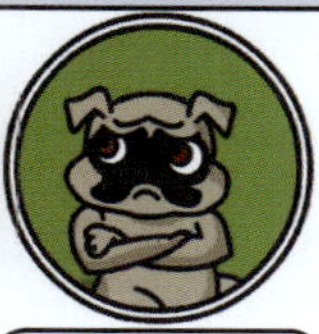

*"Sulk-Dog"*
**Sulfadoxine**

# ANTIEPILEPTICS

**Indications for antiepileptics:** epilepsy, epileptic seizures, bipolar disorder, mood disorders, neuropathic pain.

**EPILEPSY** is a neurological disorder characterized by the presence of two or more unprovoked seizure attacks due to abnormal brain discharge activity. Unfortunately, the exact cause behind this pathology still remains unknown, but it is hypothesized that epilepsy in children is correlated to congenital brain disturbances such as cerebral palsy, infection, or chromosomal abnormalities, while epilepsy in adults may be caused by aging, stroke, brain tumors, or trauma.

There are three main types of seizures: general, partial, and absence.

General seizures usually present with severe convulsions. In both general and in absence seizures there is an unsynchronized neuronal discharge involving the entire brain that is accompanied by a loss of consciousness. Partial seizures only involves one specific area of the brain, although the level of consciousness may vary from one person to another.

Treatment is usually unnecessary unless the seizure attacks are prolonged or recurrent. In such case, anticonvulsants may be warranted. Drugs used for the treatment of seizures include sodium and calcium channel blockers, gamma-aminobutyric acid (GABA) receptor enhancers, N-methyl-D-aspartate (NMDA) receptor blockers, carbonic anhydrase inhibitors, and benzodiazepines.

## Generalized (Tonic-Clonic) and Partial Seizures

***Carbamazepine*** and ***phenytoin*** are the drugs of choice for generalized and partial seizures, however they are not effective against absence seizure. These drugs bind to the surface of voltage gated sodium channels located on the surface of neurons, thereby preventing the uncontrolled firing of action potentials to adjacent cells.

***Lamotrigine*** is a sodium channel blocker, but it additionally exhibits antagonistic effects on calcium channels and 5-HT3 receptors. This prevents the release of the neurotransmitter called glutamate, which contributes to the excessive firing of electrical impulses in the brain.

***Valproate*** (sodium valproate) blocks sodium channels, and acts by increasing the level of an inhibitory neurotransmitter called GABA in the brain, either by inhibiting the enzymes responsible for its metabolism or by preventing its reuptake by neuronal cells.

***Tiagabine*** is a GABA reuptake inhibitor and produces its anti-convulsive effects by blocking the Gaba-Transporter-1 (GAT-1) receptor.

***Topiramate*** acts by blocking voltage gated sodium channels, enhancing GABA activity, and antagonizing glutamate receptors. Side effects include metabolic acidosis, closed angle glaucoma, and congenital malformations.

***Levetiracetam*** is used to treat epilepsy but its mechanism of action is not fully understood. It is believed to inhibit presynaptic calcium channels leading to a reduction in synaptic transmission.

***Gabapentin*** and ***vigabatrin*** are said to be the analogues of GABA as they resembles the molecular structure of this inhibitory neurotransmitter. For gabapentin, there are also sodium and calcium channel blocking effects and are able to prevent the formation of neuronal synapses.

***Phenobarbital*** is an effective intravenous drug which falls under the category of barbiturates. It is mainly used to treat status epilepticus and anxiety. Phenobarbital must be used with precaution as it has a narrow therapeutic window and can easily lead to overdose. The consequences can be fatal due to its ability to cause respiratory depression.

## Absence Seizures

Absence seizures are generally managed by administering ***ethosuximide*** or ***valproate***. Ethosuximide remains as the first line treatment for this form of seizure due to its approved safety profile and lack of severe side effects such as hepatotoxicity that is exhibited by its counterpart, valproate.

## Status Epilepticus

Status epilepticus is a prolonged generalized convulsion that can be fatal if not intervened promptly. As a general rule, they are treated with IV benzodiazepines such as lorazepam and diazepam, and if symptoms don't improve, IV ***phenytoin*** is often given. As mentioned above, ***phenobarbital*** can be used to treat status epilepticus, however, it would not be first line.

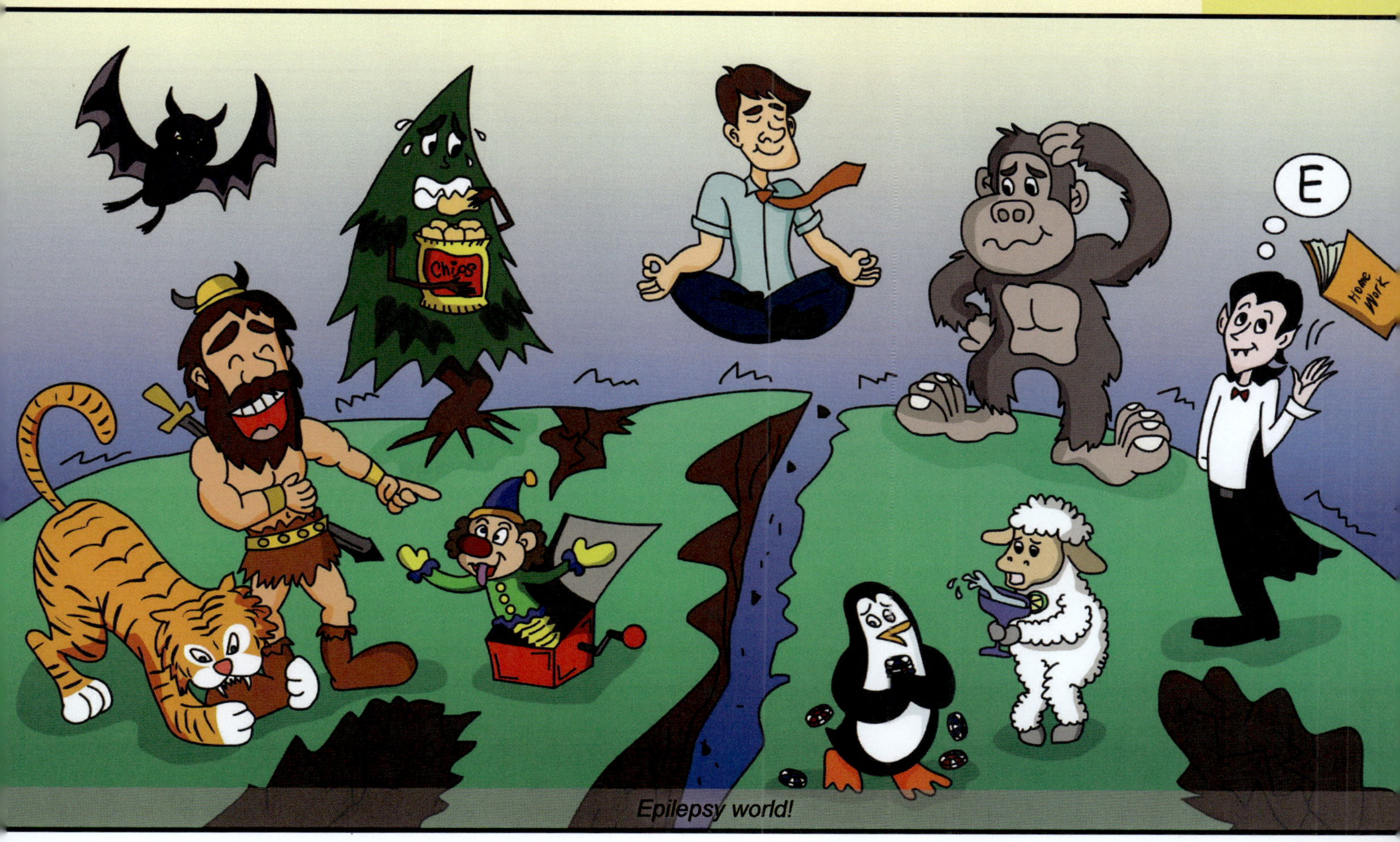

Epilepsy world!

## ANTIEPILEPTICS

👉 *The shaking earth reminds you this picture is about epilepsy! [representing the jerky movements seen in tonic-clonic seizures]*

### Generalized (Tonic-Clonic) and Partial Seizures

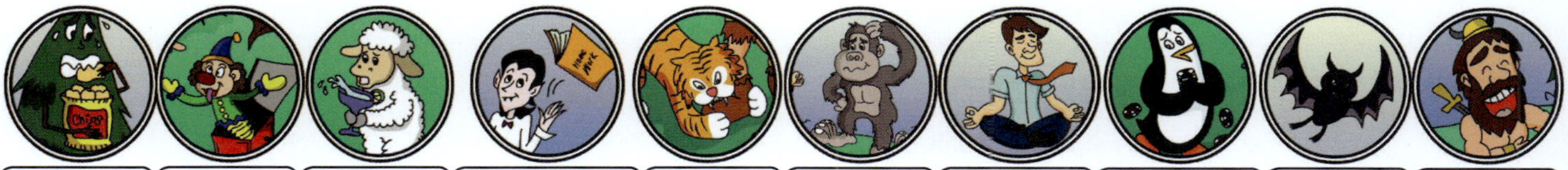

| | | | | | | | | | |
|---|---|---|---|---|---|---|---|---|---|
| "Carb-Pine" Carbamazepine | "Funny-Toy" Phenytoin | "Lamb-Gin" Lamotrigine | "Vampire-Procrastinate" Valproate | "Tiger-Bite" Tiagabine | "Toe-Primate" Topiramate | "Levitating-Man" Levetiracetam | "Gambling-Penguin" Gabapentin | "Vile-Bat" Vigabatrin | "Funny-Barbarian" Phenobarbital |

### Absence Seizures

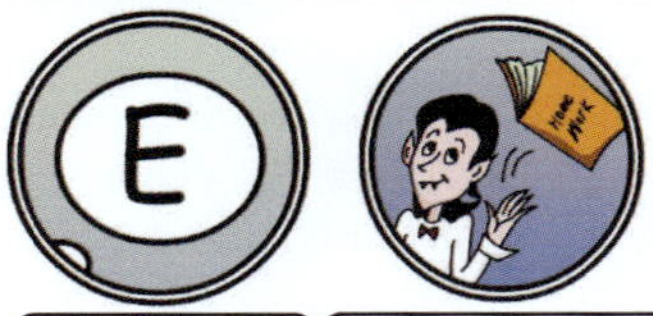

"E-Thought" Ethosuximide

"Vampire-Procrastinate" Valproate

### Status Epilepticus

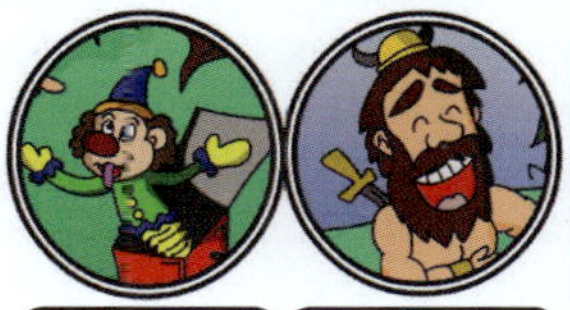

"Funny-Toy" Phenytoin

"Funny-Barbarian" Phenobarbital

** Also note benzodiazepines are used - see chapter on anxiolytics and hypnotics **

# NEUROMUSCULAR DRUGS

**Indications for neuromuscular medications:** muscular disorders, myasthenia gravis, among others.

**THE TRANSMISSION OF AN ACTION POTENTIAL** from a nerve ending to a muscle tissue involves a series of chemical signalling processes that occur in the neuromuscular junction. It begins with a nerve impulse through the presynaptic nerve caused by an influx of sodium and calcium ions. This leads to the docking of vesicles containing the neurotransmitter acetylcholine to the presynaptic membrane, and subsequently, its release into the synaptic cleft. Acetylcholine then binds to receptors located on the surface of the postsynaptic membrane. Depolarization occurs when the binding of acetylcholine to its receptors exceeds a threshold. The action potential generated from this causes the opening of sodium channels and a subsequent sodium influx into the muscle tissue. The end result is a contraction of the muscle tissue.

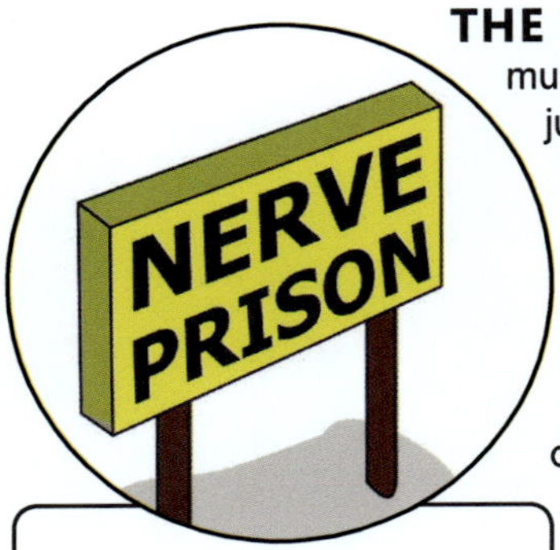


The nerve prison and muscle gate reminds you of the neuromuscular junction.

## Acetylcholinesterase Inhibitors

There are some medical conditions caused by a disorder in nerve impulse transmission that warrants the use of pharmacological treatment. For example, myasthenia gravis is an autoimmune disease that is characterized by autoimmune antibodies which target acetylcholine receptors. This leads to a clinical picture of muscle weakness. Acetylcholinesterase inhibitors are used as first line pharmacological agents. They inhibit an enzyme called acetylcholinesterase, which is an enzyme that degrades acetylcholine in the synapse. Therefore, inhibiting acetylcholinesterase leads to acetylcholine levels remaining higher for longer periods of time in the synapse. The end result is increased muscle contractility and strength. Examples of acetylcholinesterase inhibitors include ***neostigmine***, ***pyridostigmine*** and ***distigmine***.

## Reduce ACh Release

***Botulinum toxin*** is a neurotoxic protein produced by bacteria Clostridium botulinum. The toxin is lethal, however, in a controlled clinical setting it is considered safe. It is an effective treatment for overactive muscles, such as with hemifacial spasm and urinary incontinence, and is also used for cosmetic purposes to prevent the formation of wrinkles. It acts by cleaving a protein called synaptosomal-associated protein 25 (SNAP-25), preventing the fusion of acetylcholine containing vesicles to the presynaptic membrane. As a result, acetylcholine is unable to be released into the synaptic cleft via exocytosis, and paralysis occurs.

## Neuromuscular Blocking Drugs: Competitive

Competitive neuromuscular blocking drugs prevent the action of acetylcholine by binding to postsynaptic receptors. The lack of stimulation from acetylcholine will impede nerve impulse transmission and prevent muscle contraction. These drugs can be classified into depolarizing and nondepolarizing agents. The latter acts as a pure antagonist and does not generate action potential upon binding to receptors while the former will depolarize the membrane initially before inhibiting the process of depolarization.

Examples of these competitive neuromuscular blocking drugs are ***pancuronium***, ***vecuronium***, and ***rocuronium***. These drugs are used as general anesthetics and muscle relaxants, and can be used before surgical procedures to prevent muscle twitching and to aid endotracheal intubation in emergency settings. Each of these drugs have their own adverse effects and hence, the choice of drug should be tailored according to the patient's condition.

## Neuromuscular Blocking Drugs: Depolarizing

***Suxamethonium***, also known as succinylcholine, is a classic example of a depolarizing agent. The mechanism of action of suxamethonium is split into two phases. The first phase involves the opening of ion-gated channels in the ***motor end plate***, followed by depolarization caused by the release of calcium ions from the sarcoplasmic reticulum. The second phase involves desensitization of receptors at the ***nerve terminals***, making them less sensitive to acetylcholine. As there is nothing to break down suxamethonium in the synapse, the cell is unable to repolarize as the membrane potential is kept above threshold. Side effects of suxamethonium include malignant hyperthermia, hyperkalemia, and apnea.

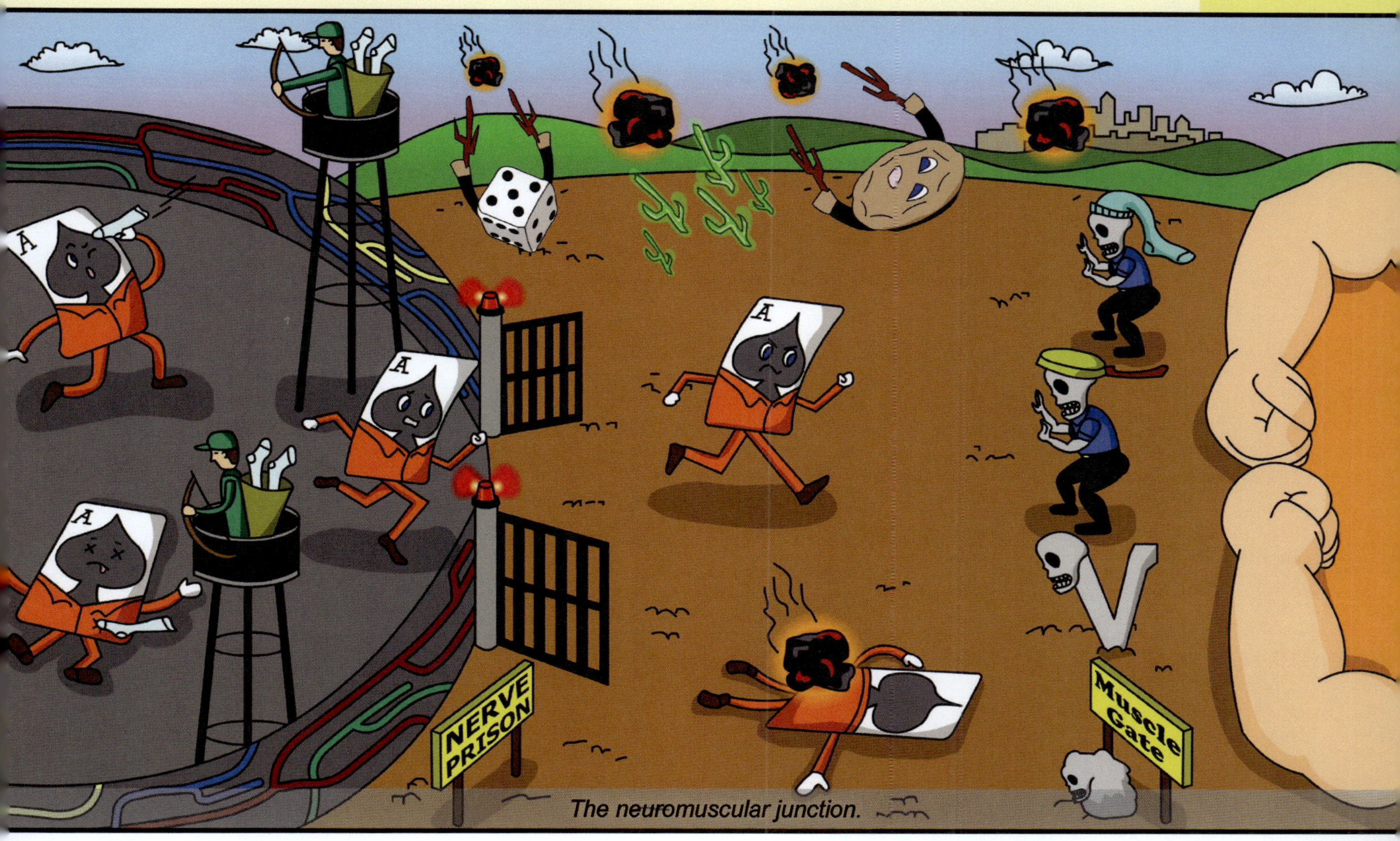

*The neuromuscular junction.*

## NEUROMUSCULAR DRUGS

☞ *The nerve prison and muscle gate reminds you of the neuromuscular junction.*

### Located at Neuro-Muscular Terminal

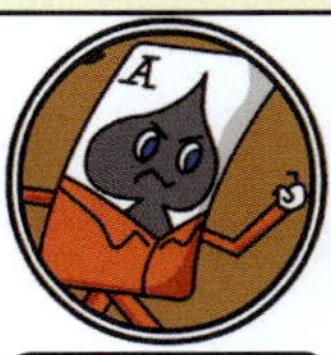
"ACE"
**Acetylcholine**

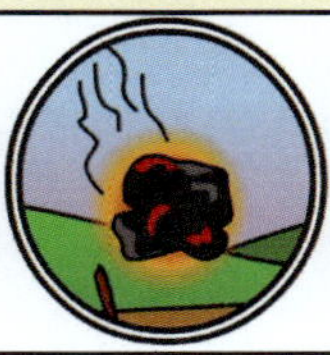
"Coal"
**Acetylcholinesterase**

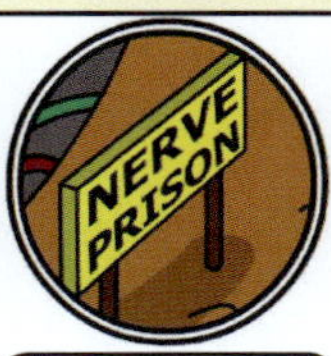

"Nerve"
**Nerve Terminal**

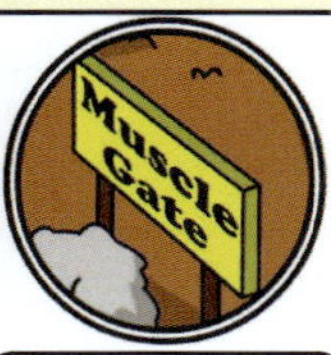

"Muscle-Gate"
**Motor End Plate**

### Acetylcholinesterase Inhibitors

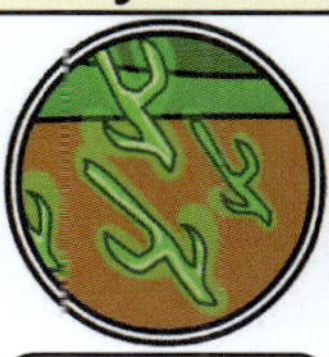
"Neon-Twig"
**Neostigmine**

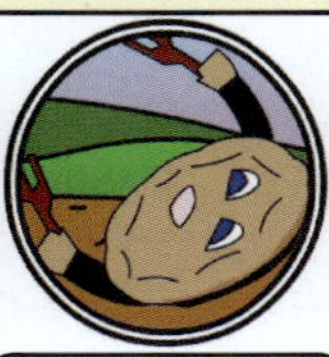
"Pie-Twig"
**Pyridostigmine**

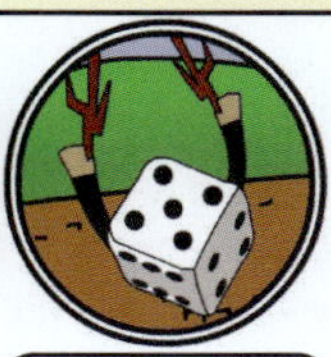
"Die-Twig"
**Distigmine**

### Reduce ACh Release

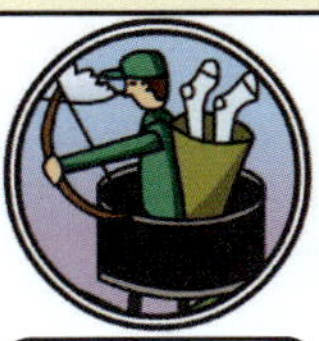
"Bow-Sox"
**Botox**

### Neuromuscular Blocking Drugs: Competitive

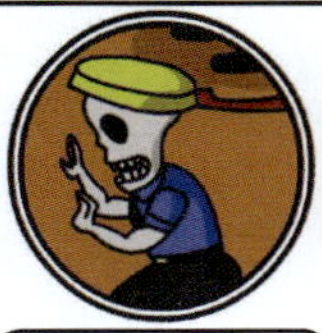
"Pan-Cranium"
**Pancuronium**

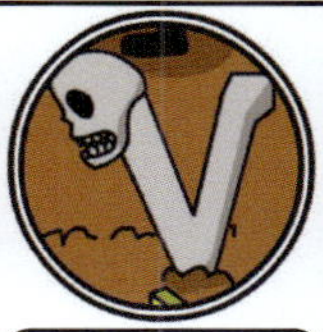
"V-Cranium"
**Vecuronium**

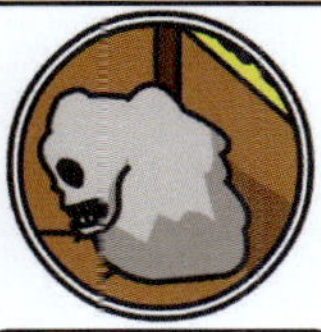
"Rock-Cranium"
**Rocuronium**

### Depolarizing

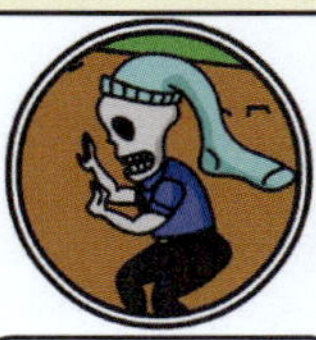
"Sock-Cranium"
**Suxamethonium**

# ANTIPARKINSON DRUGS

**Indications for Parkinson's disease medications:** Parkinson's disease.

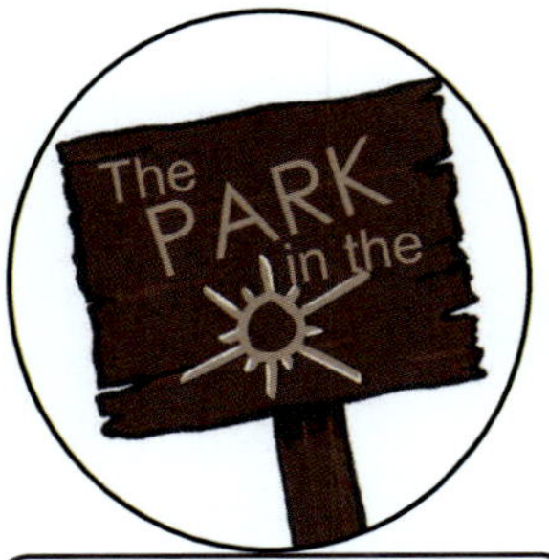


The "park in the sun" reminds you this picture is about Parkinson's disease!

**PARKINSON'S DISEASE** is a neurodegenerative disorder that affects the central nervous system (CNS), specifically destroying cells of a certain part of the brain known as substantia nigra. The disease develops gradually, causing different signs and stages. Parkinson's disease is characterized by 3 common symptoms, including tremors, dyskinesia (where voluntary muscles are rigid, stiff, and not well-controlled), and bradikynesia (slowness in movement). There is no cure for Parkinson's disease. However, there are medications to relieve symptoms, slow disease progression, and prevent complications.

## Dopamine Precursor

***Levodopa*** is a dopamine precursor that is converted inside the body by aromatic L-amino acid decarboxylase enzyme, producing dopamine. Levodopa is the first choice for treatment of Parkinson's disease, especially in older patients, and patients with bradykinesia, tremor, and rigidity.

## Peripheral Decarboxylase Inhibitor

The conversion of levodopa into dopamine affects the body not only centrally but also peripherally, causing side effects, such as orthostatic hypotension, nausea, and vomiting. In order to prevent such side effects, levodopa is combined with another substance that acts as a peripheral decarboxylase inhibitor that prevents the conversion of levodopa into dopamine in the systemic circulation. ***Carbidopa*** is an example of one of these agents.

## Dopamine Agonists

Dopamine agonists are prescribed as an adjunct or alternative therapy to levodopa. As levodopa is possibly associated with an exacerbated-degeneration of dopaminergic neurons and dopamine agonists are likely to cause less motor fluctuations, dopamine agonists are preferred in patients younger than 60 years. Below is a list of dopamine agonists divided into 3 categories:

### *Ergot Derivatives*

Ergot derivatives, such as ***bromocriptine*** and ***cabergoline***, mimic the effects of dopamine through selectively binding to dopamine D2-like receptors in the corpus striatum, inhibiting adenyl cyclase enzyme, and decreasing the intracellular concentration of cAMP. In addition, cabergoline has neuroprotective effects. Ergot derivatives decrease prolactin secretion.

### *Non-Ergot Derivatives*

***Ropinirole*** and ***pramipexole*** act similarly to bromocriptine and cabergoline, with further binding to dopamine receptors D3 and D2. Importantly, dosing of non-ergot derivatives needs to be adjusted for patients with end-stage renal failure, as these drugs are primarily excreted through the kidney. Side effects include hallucinations, feeling light-headed, shortness of breath, an increase in libido, and behavioral changes.

### *NMDA-Type Glutamate Receptor Antagonists*

***Amantadine*** has milder side effects compared to most other Parkinson medications. Although the exact mechanism of action is not well understood, it is believed to increase dopamine concentration in the CNS by inhibiting dopamine reuptake and stimulating dopamine receptors.

## Catechol-O-Methyltransferase (COMT) Inhibitors

COMT inhibitors, such as ***entacapone***, are given with levodopa to increase the effectiveness and duration of action of levodopa, as they prevent the breakdown of levodopa by COMT enzymes in the peripheral nervous system. Entacapone side effects include dyskinesia, hallucinations, confusion, nausea, and orthostatic hypotension.

## Monoamine Oxidase (MAO)-B Inhibitors

Monoamine oxidase (MAO)-B inhibitors irreversibly bind to MAO-B, and thereby prevent the metabolism of dopamine. MAO inhibitors are not advised to be used alone, and they are likely beneficial to patients at early stages of Parkinson's disease. Examples include ***selegiline*** and ***rasagiline***.

## Anticholinergics

***Benzatropine*** is an anti-cholinergic, anti-muscarinic, and anti-histaminic drug that selectively blocks the M1 muscarinic receptors located in the basal ganglia. In addition, benzatropine inhibits the presynaptic reuptake of dopamine.

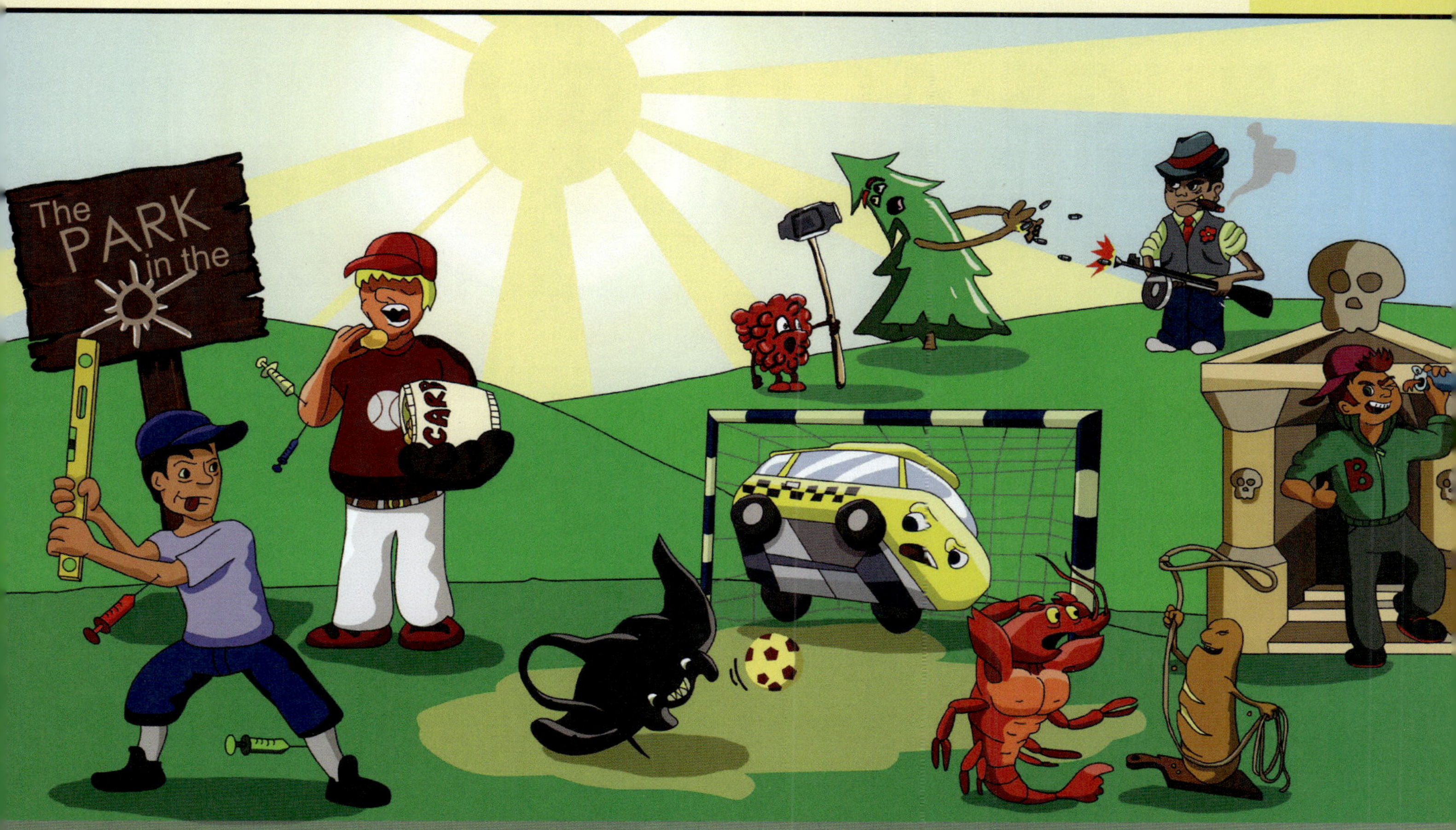


*The park in the sun!*

## PARKINSON'S DISEASE

*The "park in the sun" reminds you this picture is about Parkinson's disease!*

**D. Precursors**

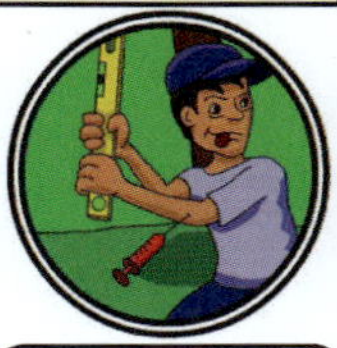

"Level-Doper"
**Levodopa**

**Decarbox. Inhib.**

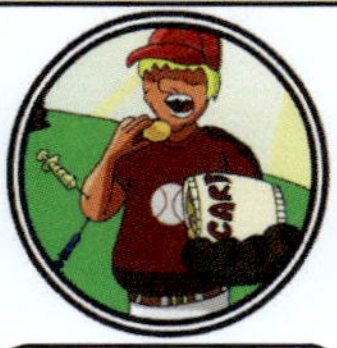

"Carb-Doper"
**Carbidopa**

**D.A.: Ergot Derivatives**

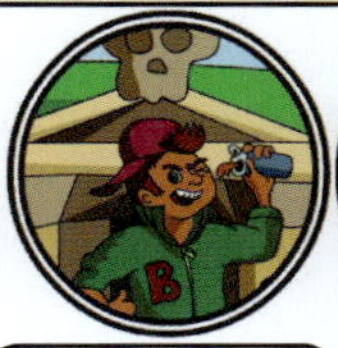

"Bro-Crypt"
**Bromocryptine**

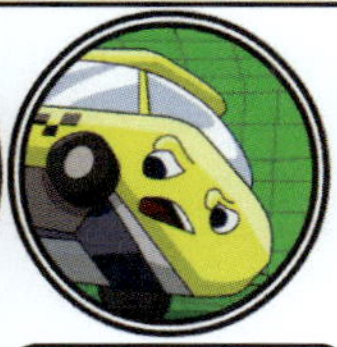

"Cab-Goalie"
**Cabergoline**

**D.A.: Non-Ergot Derivatives**

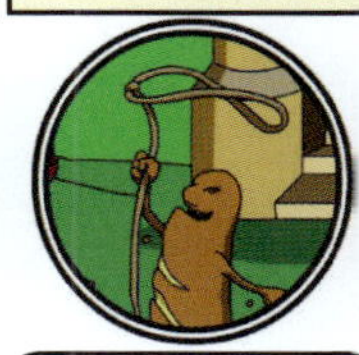

"Rope-Roll"
**Ropinirole**

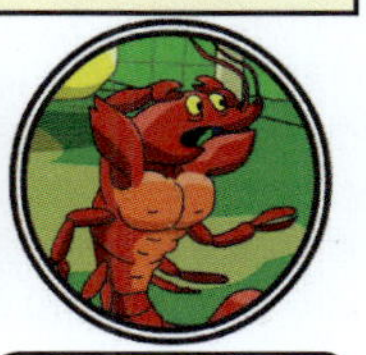

"Prawn-Pecs"
**Pramipexole**

**D.A.: Glut. Recept. Antagonist**

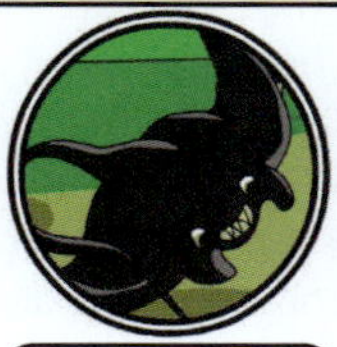

"A-Manta"
**Amantadine**

**COMT Inhibitors**

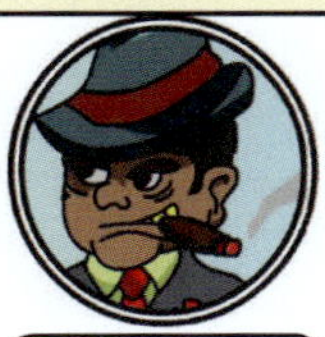

"Capone"
**Entacapone**

**MAOB Inhibitors**

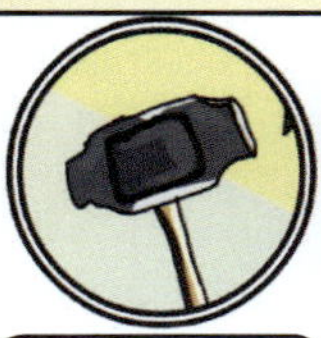

"Sledge"
**Selegiline**

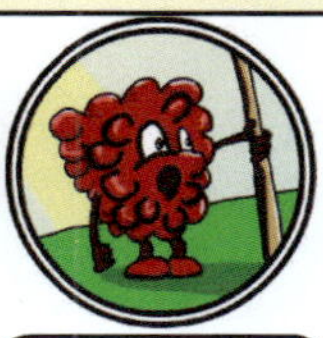

"Raspberry"
**Rasagiline**

**Anticholinergics**

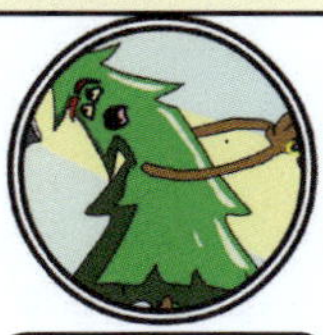

"Bent-Pine"
**Benzatropine**

# DRUGS ACTING AT CHOLINERGIC SYNAPSE

**Indications for drugs acting at cholinergic synapse:** differs between drug classes, please see below.

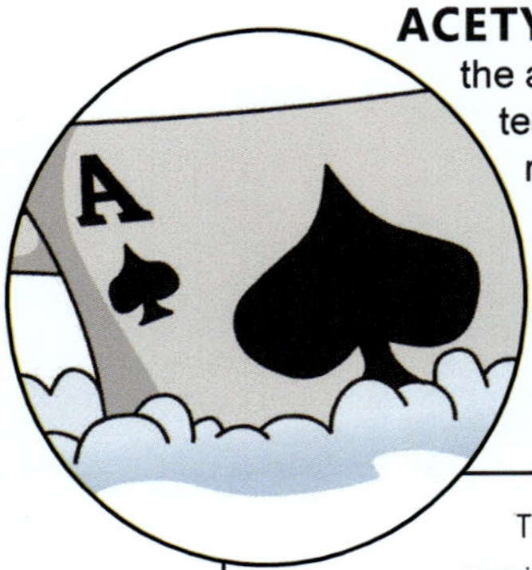


**ACETYLCHOLINE** is a neurotransmitter responsible for the transmission of chemical signaling in the autonomic nervous system. It is synthesized, stored, and released from the presynaptic nerve terminal. Acetylcholine has a wide spectrum of activity as it binds non-selectively to nicotinic receptors located in both the sympathetic and parasympathetic systems. Drugs that acts within these systems are used to treat a variety of medical conditions.

The drug class that mimics the effect of acetylcholine are called cholinomimetics.

Cholinomimetics can be sub-classified into muscarinic agonists and nicotinic agonists.

The ACE at top of picture reminds you of acetylcholine, which is the main neurotransmitter at cholinergic synapses. The characters on each field target their respective receptors, either muscarinic or nicotinic.

## Cholinomimetics: Muscarinic Agonists

***Pilocarpine*** is a muscarinic agonist used for the treatment of acute angle closure glaucoma or chronic open angle glaucoma due to increased intraocular pressure. It does so by binding to the ciliary muscle and causing it to contract. This action opens up the trabecular network and draws the aqueous humor away from the eye to relieve the built up intraocular pressure.

Another commonly used muscarinic agonist is ***bethanechol*** that binds selectively to muscarinic receptors (e.g. in bladder and gastrointestinal tract). This drug is used to treat urinary retention and to stimulate gastrointestinal movement in patients with conditions associated with decreased gastrointestinal motility.

## Cholinomimetics: Nicotinic Agonists

***Nicotine*** is an agonist that binds to nicotinic receptors. This drug stimulates a wide spectrum of physiological effects in the body including suppression of appetite and increased concentration, calmness, and metabolism. These effects are due to the stimulation of adrenergic receptors which leads to an increase in sympathetic activity.

The use of nicotine is also associated with side effects including increased risk of blood coagulation, atherosclerosis, bronchoconstriction, tremor, insulin resistance, tachycardia, and hypertension. Due to its addictive properties, controlled levels of nicotine are used therapeutically to manage nicotine dependence.

## Anti-Cholinesterases

Anti-cholinesterases do not stimulate the cholinoreceptors directly, however, they inhibit cholinesterase (an enzyme that breaks down acetylcholine), leading to a prolonged effect of acetylcholine in the synaptic cleft. This increased level of acetylcholine leads to increased neurotransmission through cholinoreceptors. Anti-cholinesterases are used for the treatment of myasthenia gravis. Examples of anti-cholinesterases include ***neostigmine***, ***pyridostigmine***, and ***edrophonium***.

## Ganglionic Blockers

Another class of drugs are those that have an antagonistic effect in the autonomic system. These drugs either block nicotinic receptors at ganglionic neurons (ganglionic blocker), or they directly inhibit the muscarinic receptors (muscarinic antagonists).

An example of a ganglionic blocker is ***trimetaphan***. Trimetaphan may be used as a second line agent in hypertensive crises or for controlled reduction of blood pressure during surgery. It binds competitively to nicotinic receptors and blocks the transmission of sympathetic and parasympathetic nervous activity.

## Muscarinic Antagonists

Muscarinic antagonists are used in a variety of medical conditions. ***Atropine*** may be used to slow down the heart rate in an emergency tachyarrhythmia and can be used as topical eye drops to temporarily inhibit the accommodation reflex and promote mydriasis. ***Benzatropine*** is a centrally acting anti-cholinergic drug effective against Parkinson's disease and dystonia. ***Scopolamine*** (hyoscine) is a antimuscarinic used to treat motion sickness and nausea.

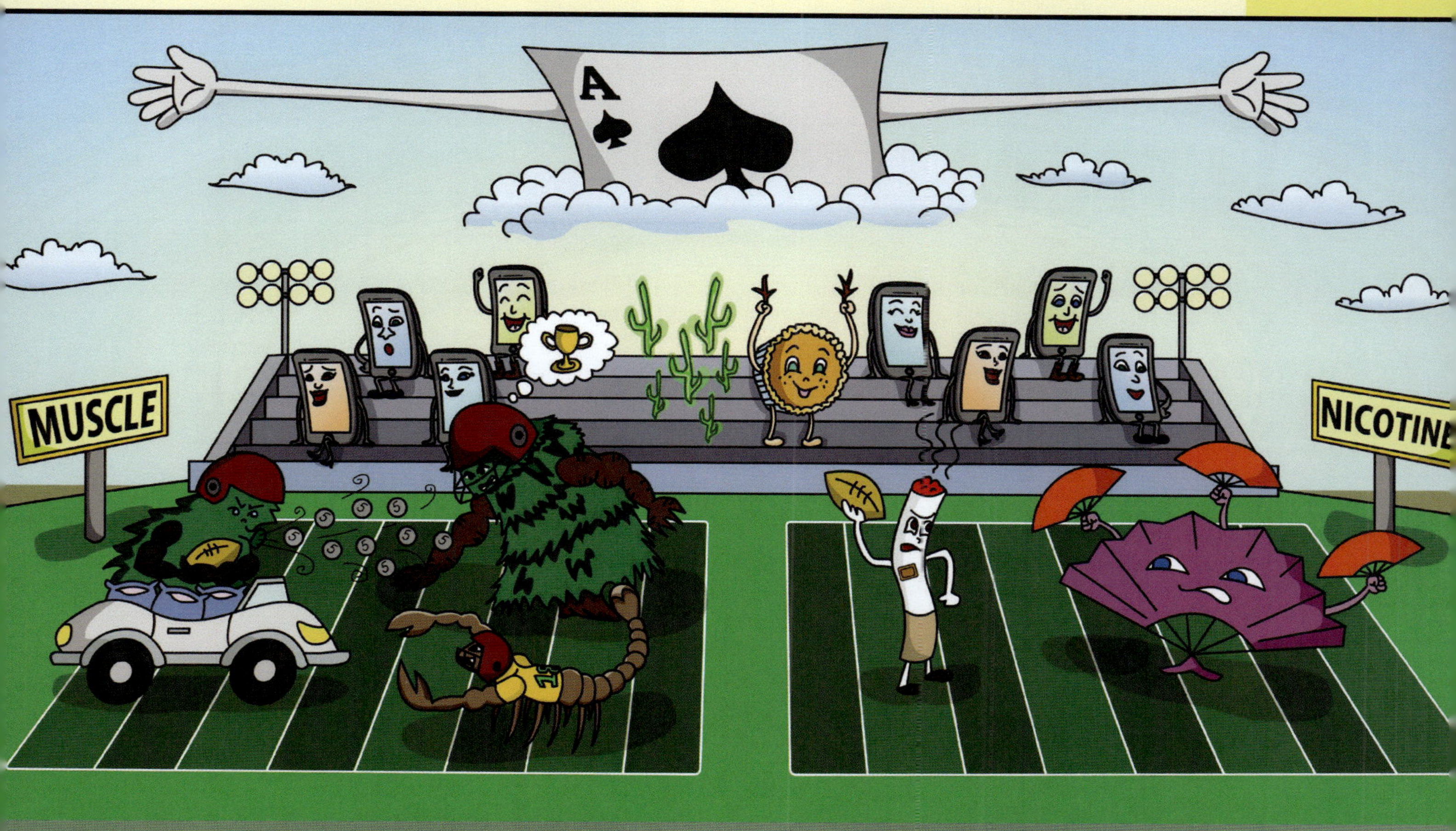


*The cholinergic games!*

## CHOLINOMIMETICS AND CHOLINERGIC RECEPTOR ANTAGONISTS

*The ACE at top of picture reminds you of acetylcholine, which is the main neurotransmitter at cholinergic synapses. The characters on each field target their respective receptors, either muscarinic or nicotinic.*

### Reminders

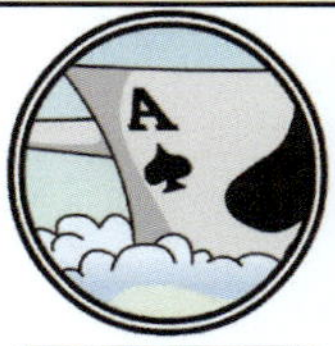


*"ACE"*
**Acetylcholine**

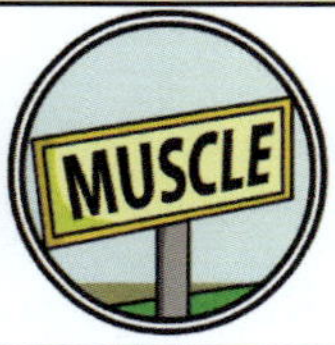


*"Muscle"*
**Muscarinic receptors**

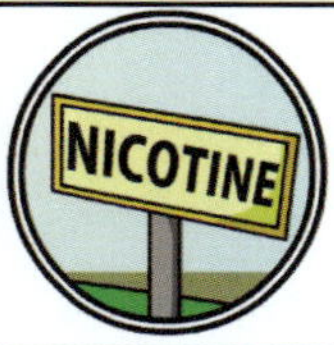


*"Nicotine"*
**Nicotinic receptors**

### Muscarinic Agonists

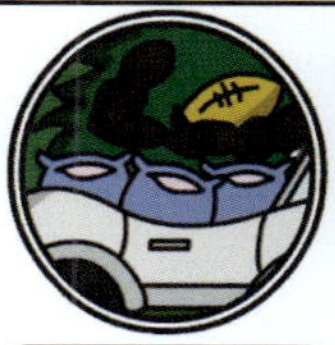

*"Pillow-Car-Pine"*
**Pilocarpine**

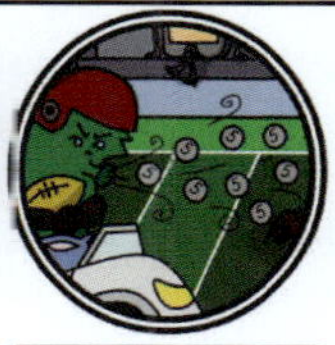

*"Breath-Nickel"*
**Bethanechol**

### Nicotinic Agonist

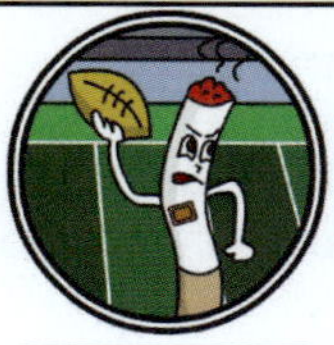

*"Nicotine [Patch]"*
**Nicotine**

### Anti-Cholinesterases

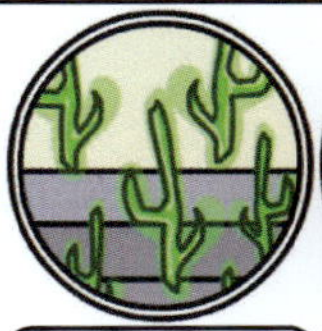

*"Neon-Twig"*
**Neostigmine**

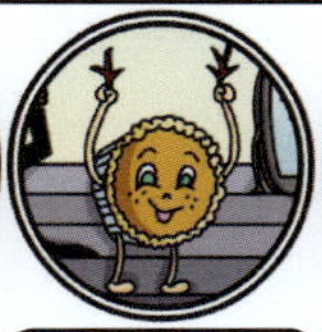

*"Pie-Twig"*
**Pyridostigmine**

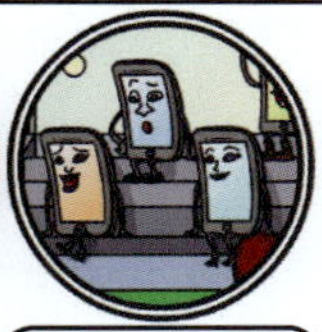

*"Row-Phones"*
**Edrophonium**

### Ganglion Blockers

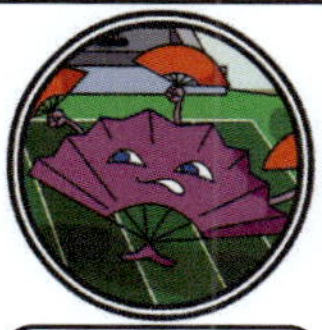

*"Tri-Fan"*
**Trimetaphan**

### Muscarinic Antagonists

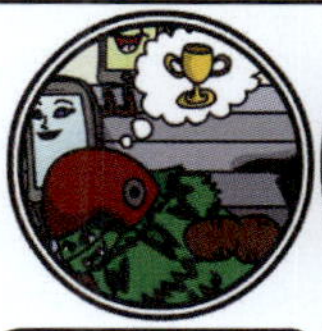

*"A-Trophy-Pine"*
**Atropine**

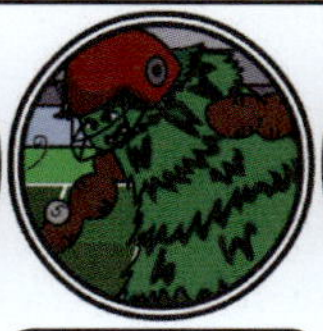

*"Bent-Pine"*
**Benzatropine**

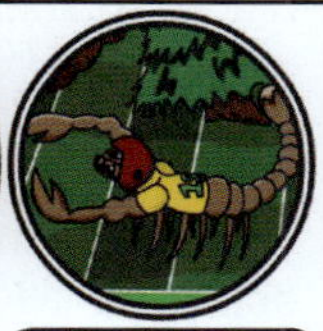

*"Scorpion"*
**Scopoamine**

# ANTIEMETICS

**Indications for antiemetic medications:** nausea and vomiting, including those associated with chemotherapy, anaesthesia, surgery, and motion sickness.

**ANTIEMETICS** are a class of drugs used to relieve nausea and vomiting caused by such things as motion sickness, gastrointestinal infections, intestinal obstruction, gastritis, pregnancy, chemotherapy, psychogenic stimuli, or disorders that increase intracranial pressure like brain tumors or hemorrhage.

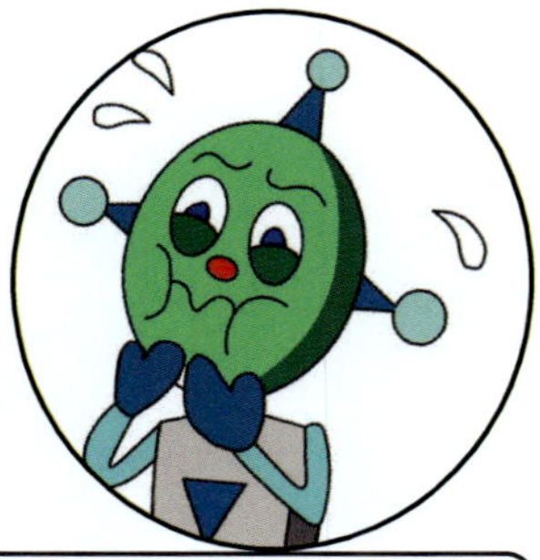

"The V Factor" [V representing vomit], along with the sick, green-faced robots, remind you this picture is about antiemetics.

Vomiting is an involuntary expulsion of stomach contents through one's mouth. In almost all cases, vomiting is preceded by nausea, an uncomfortable sensation in the abdominal region due to a gradual increase of abdominal pressure; however, in certain cases such as cholera infection, vomiting can occur without being preceded by nausea.

Nausea and vomiting can be decreased by medications through inhibition of different receptors that are located both in the brain or in the gastrointestinal tract. Within the brain, these medications target receptors in the chemoreceptor trigger zone (CTZ) of the medulla, which senses various toxins and vomiting-causing agents in the blood and cerebrospinal fluid. The CTZ then relays signals to the integrative vomiting center which causes the actions involved in vomiting.

### Histamine H1-Antagonists

Histamine H1-antagonists, such as ***promethazine*** and ***cyclizine***, are antihistamines that exhibit antiemetic and anticholinergic properties, and are usually used to prevent motion sickness and induce preoperative sedation. They prevent vomiting by blocking the H1 receptors in the CTZ and other areas of the brain. Promethazine also acts as a weak dopamine D2-receptor antagonist; therefore, a rare but important side effect includes tardive dyskinesia, a disorder characterized by repetitive and involuntary body movements. The anticholinergic property of the H1-antagonists also put patients at risk of developing prostatic hypertrophy and closed-angle glaucoma.

### 5-HT3 Receptor Antagonists

***Ondansetron*** is a 5-HT3 receptor antagonist that inhibits receptors found in the peripheral vagal nerve terminals and also in the CTZ of the area postrema. As a result, serotonin secreted by the enterochromaffin cells in the intestines will be unable to trigger a vomiting reflex through the vagal nerve. This class of drug has a good tolerability profile, but side effects may include constipation, diarrhea, and ototoxicity in severe cases.

### Dopamine D2-Receptor Antagonists

***Metoclopramide*** and ***domperidone*** are classified as dopamine D2-receptor antagonists, and are commonly used to treat medical conditions associated with nausea and delayed stomach emptying. They also appear to have a serotonin antagonism effect.

### Neurokinin Receptor Antagonists

Neurokinin receptor antagonists, such as ***aprepitant***, are used for acute and delayed chemotherapy-induced nausea and vomiting, and prevention of postoperative nausea and vomiting. It is a G-protein coupled receptor that acts by blocking signals given off by the neurokinin-1 receptors and its vomiting inducing ligand, substance P.

### Muscarinic Receptor Antagonists

Muscarinic receptor antagonists, such as ***scopolamine*** (also known as hyoscine), is used for the prevention of postoperative vomiting, and in some cases to treat vomiting induced by sea sickness. Although the mechanism of action of scopolamine is not thoroughly understood, the antiemetic property may be due to the blockage of M1-receptors found in post-ganglionic nerves of the central nervous system. Some side effects of scopolamine include dry mouth, tachycardia, skin rashes, or itchiness.

### Cannabinoids

Cannabinoids act on cannabinoid receptors in the brain. Although its exact antiemetic mechanism is not well established, it is effective for prevention of vomiting in cancer patients who are undergoing chemotherapy. An example of one of these drugs in ***nabilone***.

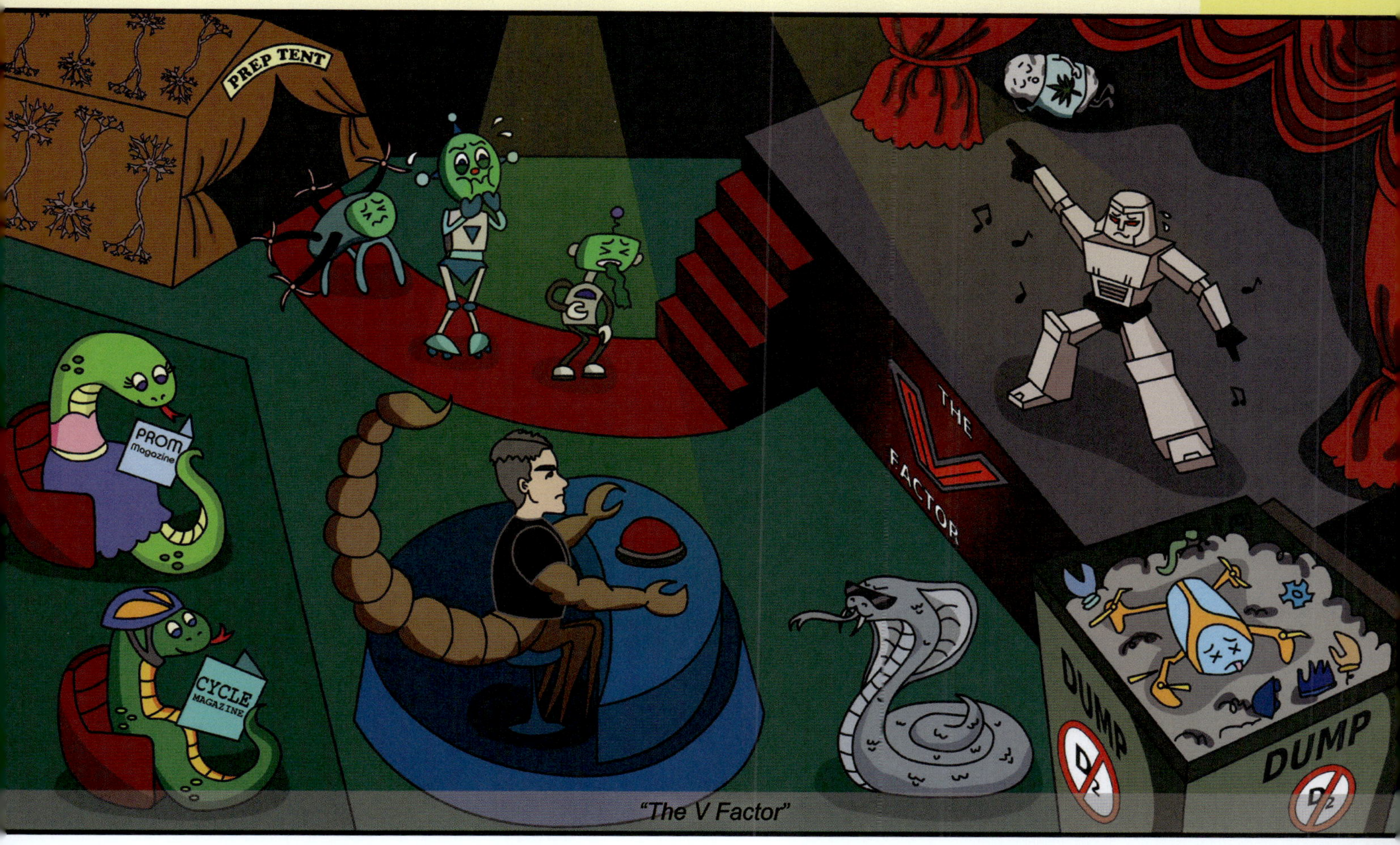


"The V Factor"

## ANTIEMETICS

👉 *"The V Factor" [V representing vomit], along with the sick, green-faced robots, remind you this picture is about antiemetics.*

### Histamine H1-Antagonists

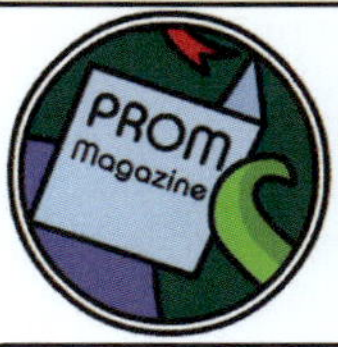


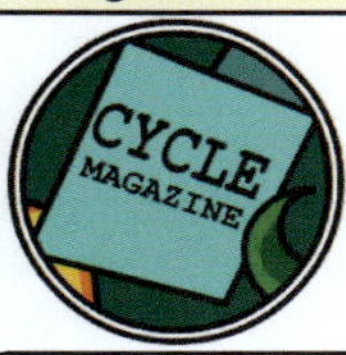


*"Prom-Magazine"*
**Promethazine**

*"Cycle-Magazine"*
**Cyclizine**

### 5-HT3-Receptor Antagonists

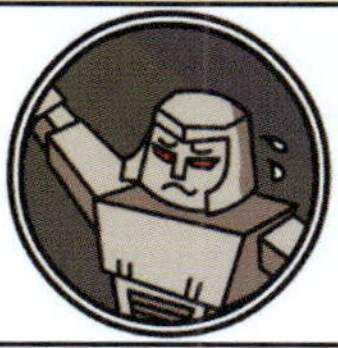

*"On[Stage]-Dancing"*
**Ondansetron**

### D2-Receptor Antagonists

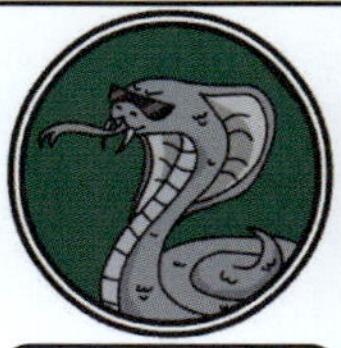

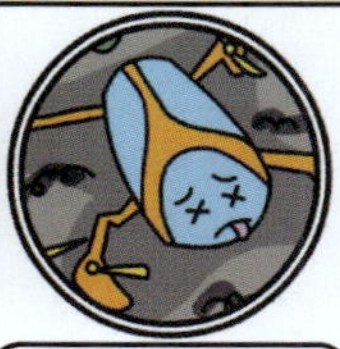

*"Metal-Cobra"*
**Metoclopramide**

*"Dump-Drone"*
**Domperidone**

### NK1 Receptor Antagonists

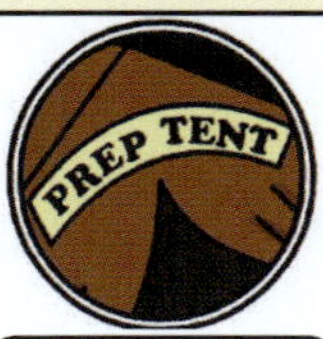


*"Prep-Tent"*
**Aprepitant**

### Muscarinic Receptor Antagonists

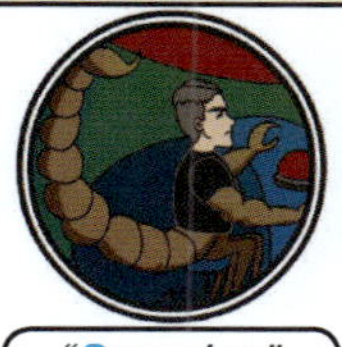

*"Scorpion"*
**Scopolamine**

### Cannabinoids

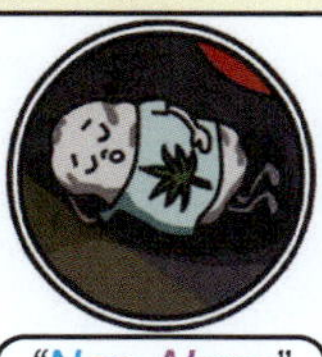

*"Nap-Alone"*
**Nabilone**

# ANTIDEPRESSANTS

**Indications for antidepressant medications:** depression, anxiety disorders, OCD, panic disorders, PTSD.

**MAJOR DEPRESSIVE DISORDER (MDD)** is characterized by low mood, loss of interest or pleasure, and low energy for a prolonged period of time. Symptoms include sleep disturbances, guilt, poor concentration, change in appetite, psychomotor agitation or retardation, and thoughts of suicide. Pharmacological treatments are described below.

## Selective Serotonin Reuptake Inhibitors (SSRIs)

The most commonly prescribed class of antidepressants are the selective serotonin reuptake inhibitors (SSRIs). Examples include ***fluoxetine***, ***paroxetine***, ***citalopram***, and ***sertraline***. As the name suggests, SSRIs prevent the reuptake of serotonin back into the presynaptic terminal by blocking serotonin transporters (SERT). As a result, more serotonin will be available to bind at the postsynaptic receptors.

Besides MDD, SSRIs are also proven to be effective for the treatment of post-traumatic stress and anxiety disorders, however, the use of SSRIs are not without their side effects. Reported drug adverse effects include decreased libido, restlessness, diarrhoea, nausea, and suicidal tendency.

## Serotonin Noradrenaline Reuptake Inhibitors (SNRIs)

Serotonin noradrenaline reuptake inhibitors (SNRIs) act mainly on both SERT and norepinephrine transporters (NET), leading to an increase in both serotonin and norepinephrine in the synaptic cleft. Examples include ***duloxetine*** and ***venlafaxine***, and common side effects are nausea, dizziness, and sweating. Duloxetine has also been shown to help symptoms of chronic pain, and therefore is often prescribed for those with a combination of depression and chronic pain. Venlafaxine is often prescribed for those who have depression and lethargy, as it can increase energy and wakefulness.

## Tricyclic Antidepressants (TCAs)

Tricyclic antidepressants (TCAs) examples include ***amitriptyline***, ***imipramine***, ***lofepramine,*** and ***dosulepin***. Along with MDD, TCAs are also effective in the treatment of other psychiatric disorders such as generalized anxiety disorder, obsessive compulsive disorder, and panic attacks. The antidepressants act by inhibiting the reuptake of serotonin and norepinephrine through blocking SERT and NET, and antagonize other types of receptors such as the alpha-1 adrenergic receptors, NMDA receptors, histamine receptors, and cholinergic muscarinic receptors.

TCAs can cause a wide spectrum of side effects such as constipation, decrease in bowel movements, urinary retention, dry mouth, hypotension, and tachycardia. The use of TCAs in clinical practice has been decreasing over the years due to these side effects and has been largely replaced by newer classes of drugs, like SSRIs.

## Serotonin Antagonist and Reuptake Inhibitors (SARIs)

***Trazodone*** is classified as a serotonin antagonist and reuptake inhibitor (SARI). Besides depression, it can also be used to treat anxiety disorders and insomnia.

## Monoamine Oxidase Inhibitors (MAOIs)

Monoamine oxidase inhibitors (MAOIs) have long been used for the treatment of major depression, however, due to their high side effect profile and the success of electroconvulsive therapy, MAOI use has decreased substantially. Examples include ***phenelzine***, ***moclobemide***, and ***isocarboxazid***.

MAOIs act by irreversibly binding to monoamine oxidase (classified into MAO-A and MAO-B), an enzyme responsible for metabolizing monoamine neurotransmitters. MAO-A degrades three monoamines: serotonin, norepinephrine, and dopamine, while MAO-B only degrades dopamine. Therefore, MAOI inhibitors used for depression involve inhibiting MAO-A (usually a non-selective MAOI), whereas selective MAO-B inhibitors are used for treating Parkinson's disease (due to its selective effects on dopamine).

MAOIs are famous for being able to bring about a hypertensive crisis. As MAO-A and B degrade tyramine (found in foods like fine wines and cheeses), if large amounts of tyramine are eaten while on a MAOI, catecholamines build up and lead to blood vessel constriction, which in turn can lead to dangerously high blood pressure.

## Noradrenergic and Specific Serotonergic Antidepressants (NaSSA)

Antidepressants that blocks the alpha-2 adrenergic receptors and 5-HT2 serotonin receptors in the central nervous system are called noradrenergic and specific serotonergic antidepressants (NaSSA). An example includes ***mirtazapine***, often used for elderly patients, as side effects can help sleep and increased appetite.

## Norepinephrine Reuptake Inhibitor (NRI)

Norepinephrine reuptake inhibitors (NRIs), such as ***reboxetine*** strongly inhibits the NET and minorly inhibits SERT. Effectiveness of this medication is still under investigation.

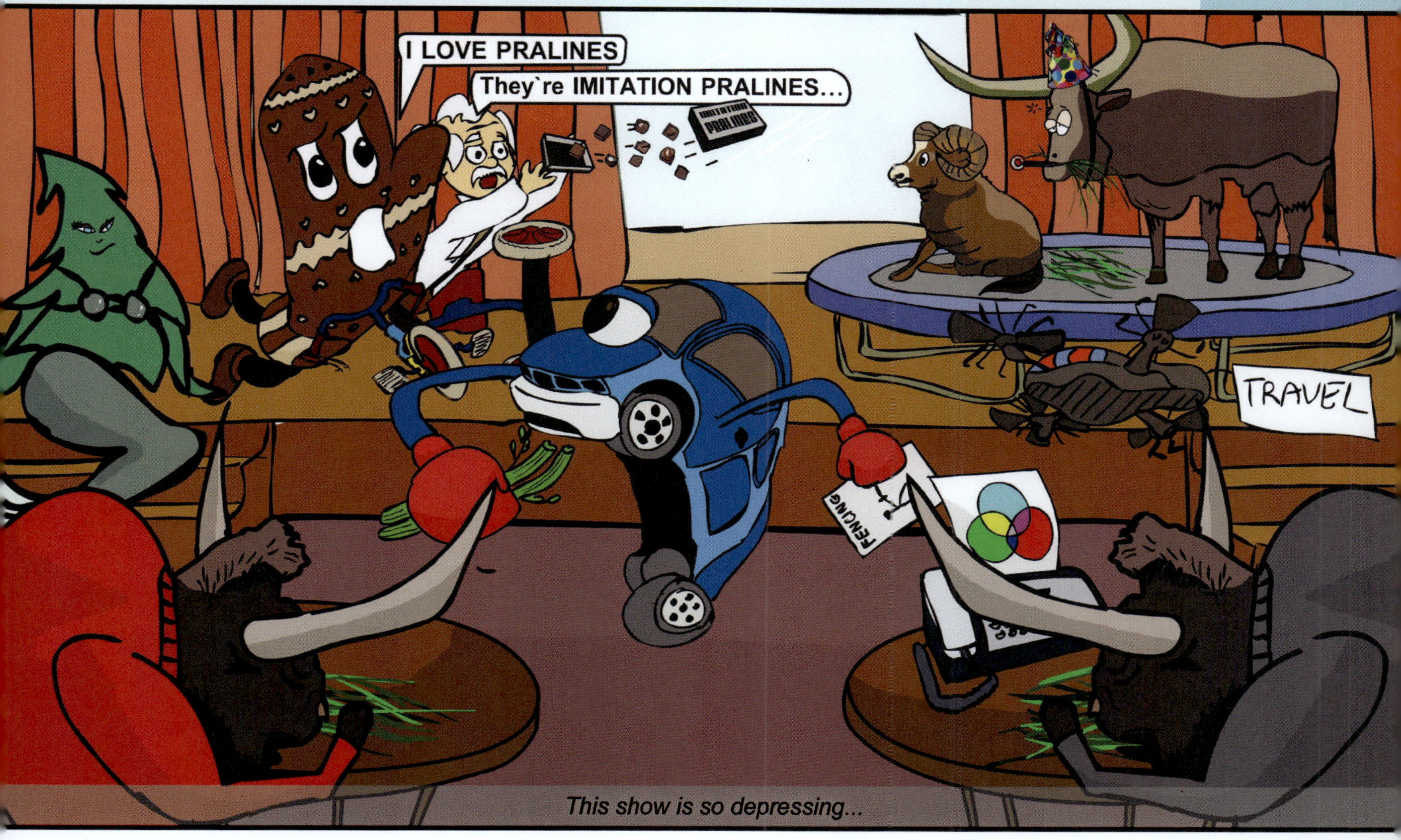
I LOVE PRALINES
They're IMITATION PRALINES...
IMITATION PRALINES
TRAVEL
FENCING
This show is so depressing...

## ANTIDEPRESSANTS

*The depressed oxen on bottom of picture remind you this picture is about depression.*

### SSRIs

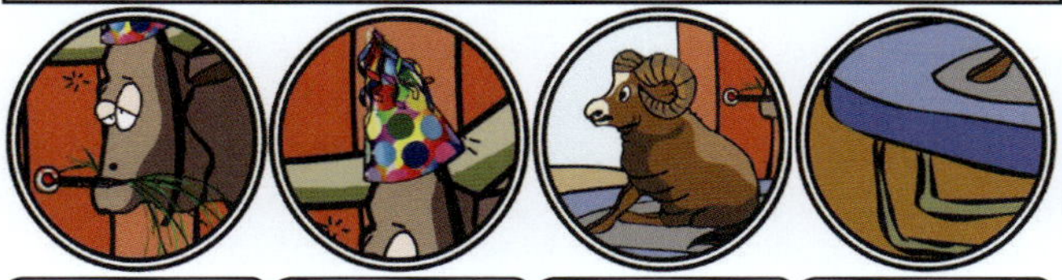

| "Flu-Ox" | "Party-Ox" | "Sitting-Ram" | "Trampoline" |
|---|---|---|---|
| **Fluoxetine** | **Paroxetine** | **Citalopram** | **Sertraline** |

### SNRIs

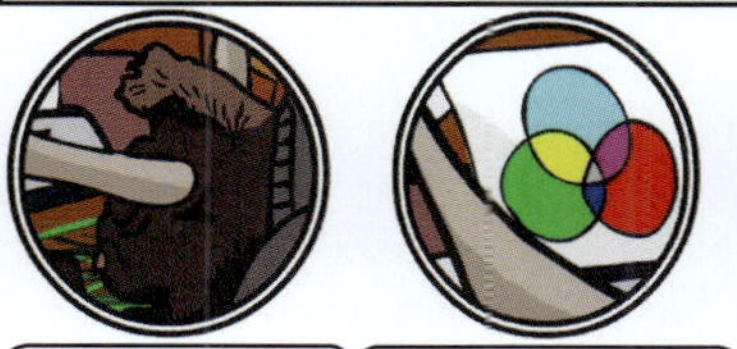

| "Dull-Ox-Eating" | "Ven[diagram]-Faxing" |
|---|---|
| **Duloxetine** | **Venlafaxine** |

### NaSSA

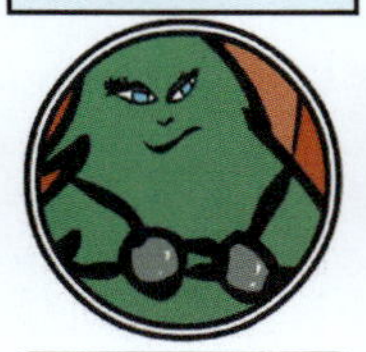

"Mermaid-Pine"
**Mirtazapine**

### NRI

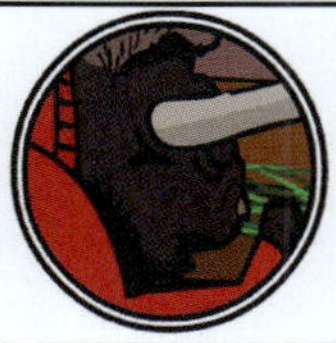

"Red-Ox-Eating"
**Reboxetine**

### TCAs

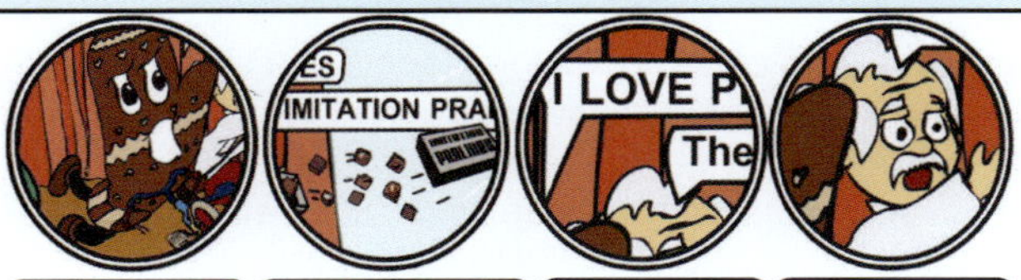

| "A-Mitt-Trip" | "Imitation-Praline" | "Love-Praline" | "Doc-Loopy" |
|---|---|---|---|
| **Amitriptyline** | **Imipramine** | **Lofepramine** | **Dosulepin** |

### SARI

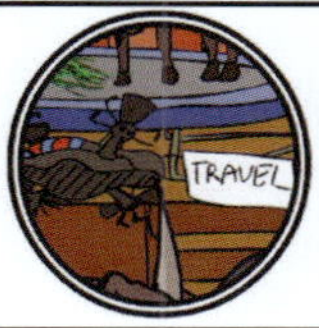

"Travel-Drone"
**Trazodone**

### MAOIs

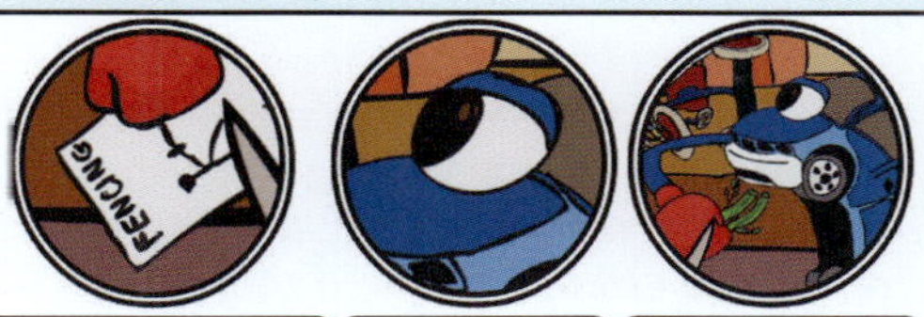

| "Fencing-Magazine" | "Mono-Eye" | "Eye-Car-Box" |
|---|---|---|
| **Phenelzine** | **Moclobemide** | **Isocarboxazid** |

# ANTIPSYCHOTICS

**Indications for antipsychotic medications:** psychosis, schizophrenia, bipolar disorder.

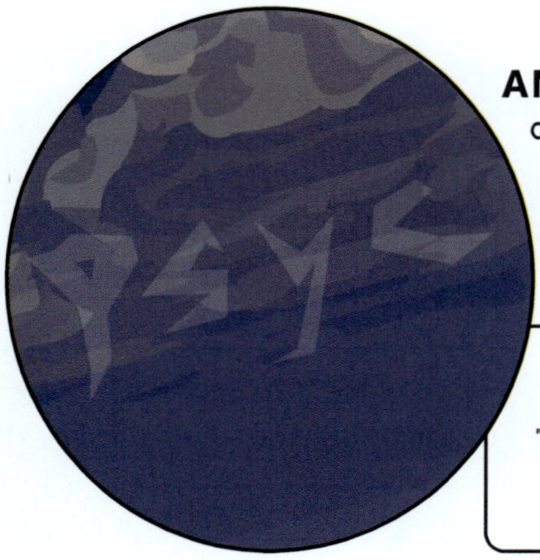


**ANTIPSYCHOTICS** are a class of drugs that are used for the treatment of psychotic disorders including psychosis, schizophrenia, and bipolar disorder. They are split into first and second generation classes. These medications are usually given orally or intramuscularly (IM). Some are given as an depot IM injection for continued slow release and gradual absorption.

The word in the clouds saying "psyc" reminds you this picture is about antipsychotics.

## First Generation Antipsychotics (FGAs)

First generation antipsychotics (FGAs) have tendencies to cause more extrapyramidal side effects (EPS) than second generation antipsychotics (SGAs). EPS include acute dystonia, akathisia, akinesia, and tardive dyskinesia.

***Chlorpromazine*** is a classic representation of a FGA, and the first antipsychotic on the market. It acts by blocking D2 dopamine receptors in the brain which subsequently decreases dopaminergic neurotransmission. Along with antipsychotic properties, chlorpromazine is also used for other indications, such as to relieve nausea and vomiting, and to treat intractable hiccups.

***Fluphenazine*** is a low potency FGA that blocks both D1 and D2 receptors. Fluphenazine is typically only used for psychosis, including schizophrenia. However, with introduction of newer SGAs, its usage has decreased substantially.

***Haloperidol*** is another example of a FGA and is considered to have a higher potency than other members of the drug class. As a result, adverse effects from haloperidol use may be more common and severe, with examples including neuroleptic malignant syndrome and QT prolongation. This drug is often used in hospitals for acutely delirious or agitated patients.

## Second Generation Antipsychotics (SGAs)

SGAs tend to cause more metabolic side effects than FGAs, such as weight gain, diabetes, and hypercholesterolemia.

***Clozapine*** was the first SGA introduced into the market. The mechanism of action of clozapine involves binding and blocking serotonin and dopamine receptors in the brain, ultimately decreasing dopaminergic neurotransmission. Although considered the most effective antipsychotic, clozapine is not first line therapy due to the chance of agranulocytosis, a dangerous leukopenia, and is usually only used in individuals that have failed to respond to at least two other antipsychotics. Furthermore, high clozapine levels in the blood have been associated with cardiac toxicity. For these reasons, patients treated with clozapine must be monitored with regular blood tests including full blood counts and clozapine levels.

Other SGAs include ***asenapine***, ***olanzapine***, ***quetiapine***, ***ziprasidone***, ***risperidone***, ***aripiprazole***, ***lurasidone***, and ***paliperidone***. SGAs block dopamine receptors in the brain, leading to decreased dopaminergic neurotransmission. All of these drugs may differ in chemical structures and biochemical properties, and the side effects may also vary from one patient to another. For example, olanzapine is considered the most effective SGA, bar clozapine, but carries a high metabolic side effect profile compared to the other SGAs.

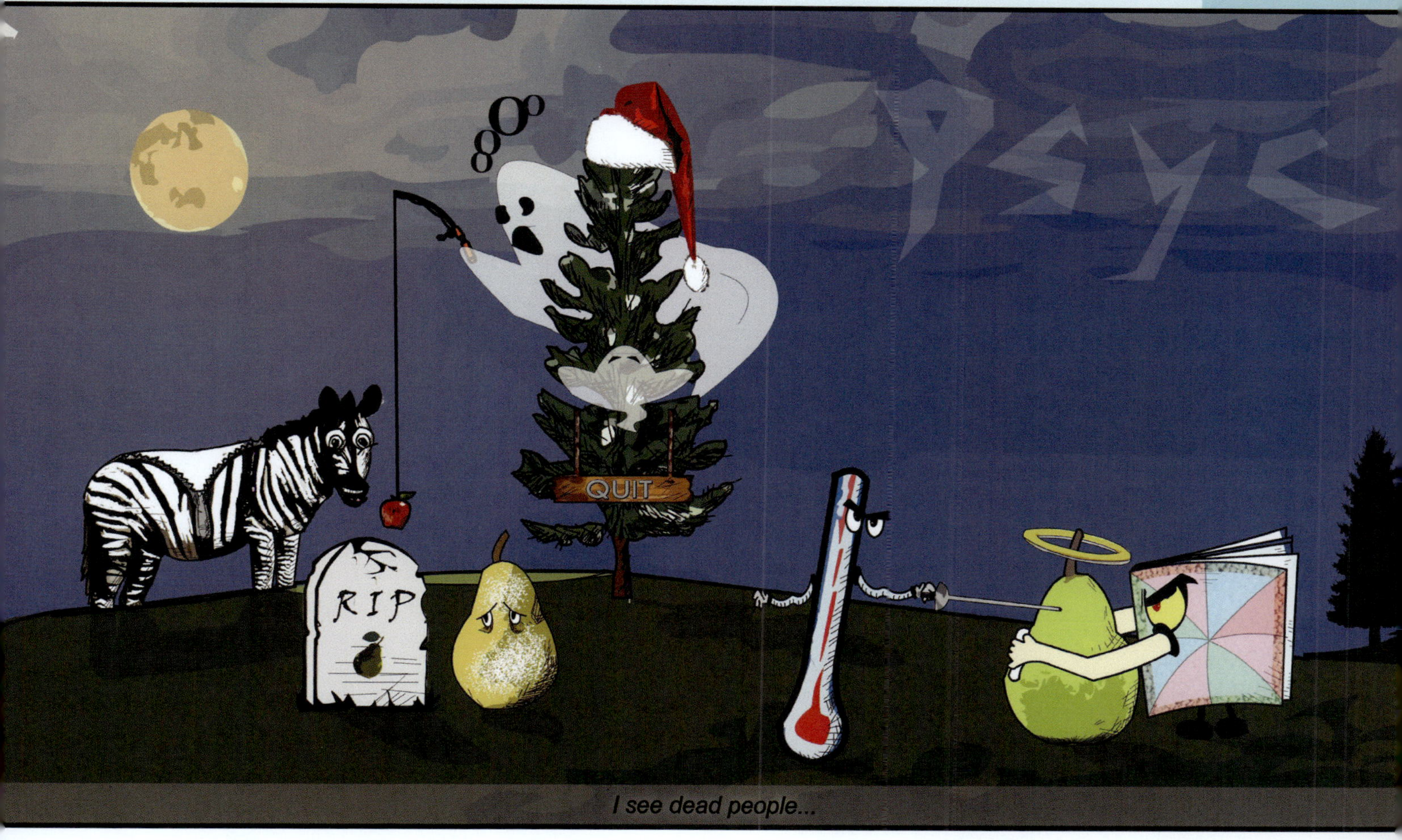


## ANTIPSYCHOTICS

The word in the clouds saying "psyc" reminds you this picture is about psychiatry.

### First Generation Antipsychotics Typical Neurolepnes .

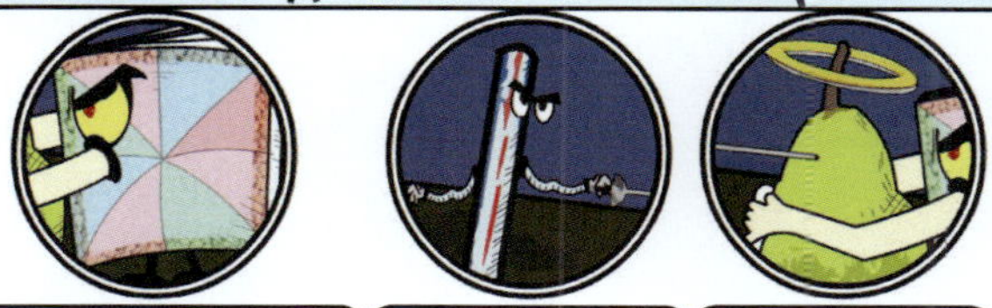

| | | |
|---|---|---|
| *"Colorful-Magazine"* **Chlorpromazine** | *"Flu-Fencing"* **Fluphenazine** | *"Ha'o-Pear"* **Haloperidol** |

Phenothiazines — Butyrophenone

### Second Generation Antipsychotics

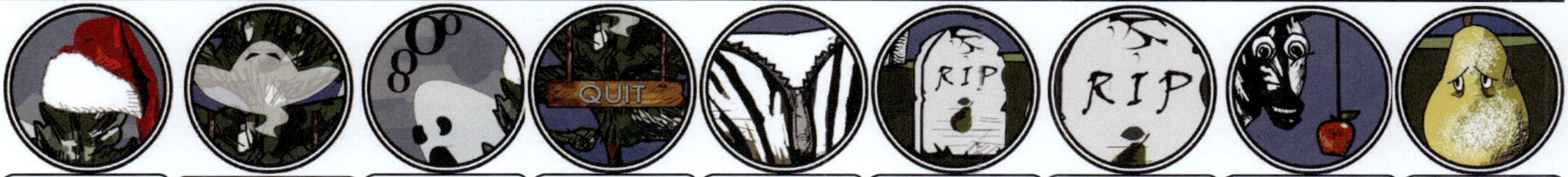

| | | | | | | | | |
|---|---|---|---|---|---|---|---|---|
| *"Clause-Pine"* **Clozapine** | *"Ascention-Pine"* **Asenapine** | *"O-Pine"* **Olanzepine** | *"Quit-Pine"* **Quetiapine** | *"Zip-Zebra"* **Ziprasidone** | *"RIP"* **Risperidone** | *"A-RIP"* **Aripiprazole** | *"Lure"* **Lurasidone** | *"Pale-Pear"* **Paliperidone** |

Atypical neuroleptic — Atypical neuroleptic

# ANXIOLYTICS & HYPNOTICS

**Indications for anxiolytics and hypnotics:** anxiety disorders, seizures, alcohol withdrawal.

**ANXIETY** is characterized by unpleasant feelings of tension, worry, and nervousness over unrealized events. The emotional changes are often accompanied by physical symptoms such as tremor, sweating, palpitations, and the inability to concentrate.

Anxiety when encountering difficult situations is considered a normal human behaviour, however, when a person experiences anxiety regularly and to the extent where their life is significantly affected, he or she may suffer from an anxiety disorder.

There is a wide range of pharmacological medications proven to be effective for the treatment of anxiety disorders, known as anxiolytics.

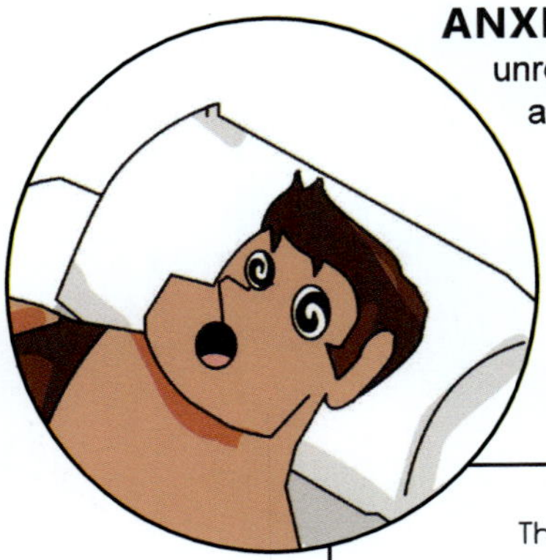

The hypnotized man reminds you this picture is about anxiolytics and hypnotics.

## Antidepressants

Although classified as antidepressants, these medications have anxiolytic effects and are often used as first line treatment in anxiety disorders.

Selective serotonin reuptake inhibitors (SSRIs), such as ***fluoxetine***, ***paroxetine,*** and ***sertraline***, treat anxiety disorders by preventing serotonin reuptake at the neuronal synapse, causing an increase of serotonin in the synaptic cleft and enhancing its effect on postsynaptic receptors.

Tricyclic antidepressants (TCAs), like ***amitriptyline***, act by inhibiting the reuptake of norepinephrine and serotonin, antagonizing acetylcholine and histamine receptors, and inhibiting sodium and calcium ion channels.

***Buspirone*** is an anxiolytic and can also augment SSRI therapy in major depression. Although the exact mechanism of action is not well understood, buspirone is thought to have an agonist effect on 5-HT1A receptors, and a mild antagonistic effect on dopamine D2 receptors.

In general, antidepressants are preferred for the treatment of anxiety over benzodiazepines because they do not have a sedative effect and do not lead to drug dependence.

## Benzodiazepines

Benzodiazepines are one of the most common classes of medication for treating anxiety disorders. They are classified according to their duration of effect. ***Lorazepam*** and ***temazepam*** are examples of shorter acting drugs, while ***diazepam*** and ***nitrazepam*** have longer durations of action. Benzodiazepines enhance the effect of gamma aminobutyric acid (GABA) in the central nervous system through the binding of the drug to the benzodiazepine modulatory receptor site located adjacent to GABA$_A$ receptors. This leads to a change in the configuration of GABA$_A$ receptors and increases the frequency of chloride channel opening in the neuron. As a result, hyperpolarization of the cells occurs leading to a neuronal inhibitory effect. This mechanism of action enables benzodiazepines to also be used as a hypnotic to treat sleep disorders. Side effects of benzodiazepine include drowsiness, impaired consciousness, loss of body movement coordination, and drug dependence.

## Z-Drugs

Z-drugs, otherwise known as nonbenzodiazepine hypnotics, are hypnotics that have similar effects to benzodiazepines and act on the same receptors. The main difference between the two classes are that they have different chemical structures. Examples of the Z-drugs include ***zopiclone***, ***zolpidem*** and ***zaleplon***.

## Beta-Blockers

Although beta-blockers such as ***propranolol*** are not first line agents in the treatment of anxiety disorders, it is effective in relieving the physical symptoms of anxiety. These symptoms are related to sympathetic overactivity and include sweating, tremor, palpitations, and tachycardia.

## Barbiturate Derivative

***Amobarbital*** is a barbiturate derivative that activates GABA$_A$ receptors by binding and increasing the duration of their chloride channel opening. The use of this agent for extended periods of time can lead to physical dependence, and on discontinuation, serious withdrawal symptoms can occur.

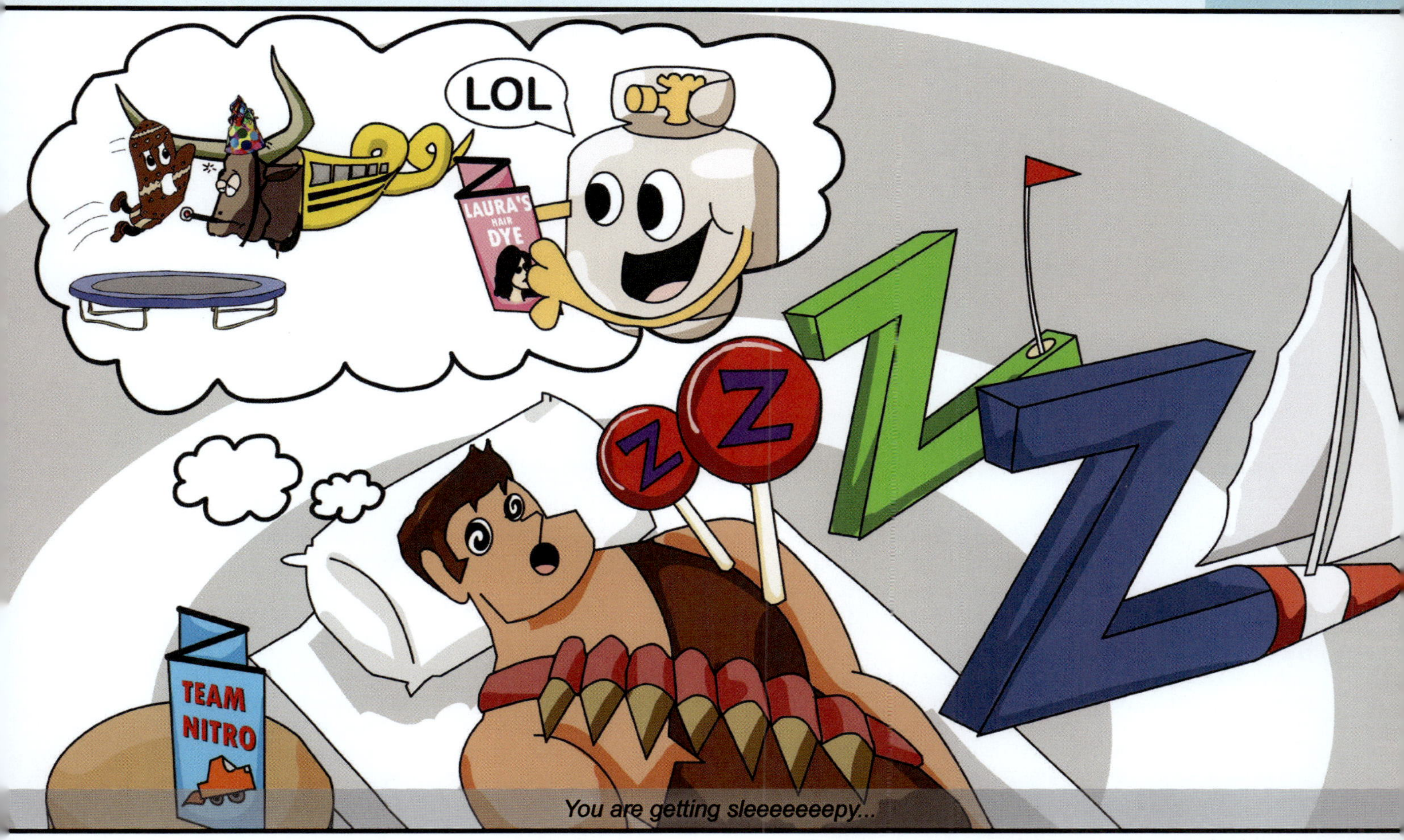


## ANXIOLYTICS & HYPNOTICS

☞ *The hypnotized man reminds you this picture is about anxiolytics and hypnotics.*

### Benzodiazepines (Short)

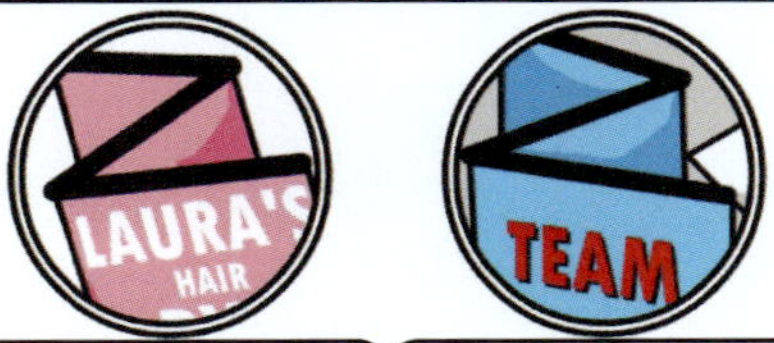


| | |
|---|---|
| *"Laura-Z-Pamphlet"* **Lorazepam** | *"Team-Z-Pamphlet"* **Temazepam** |

### Benzodiazepines (Long)

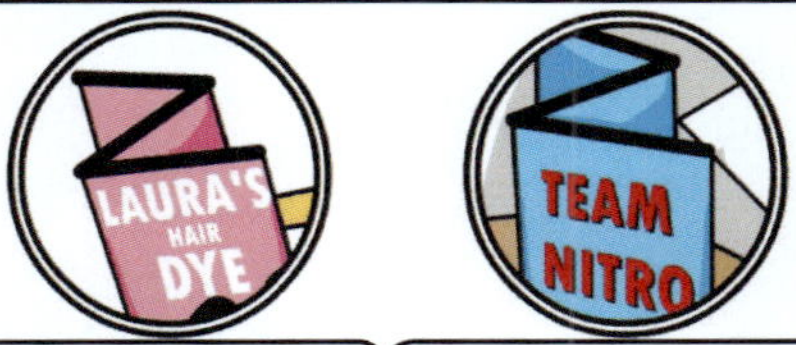


| | |
|---|---|
| *"Dye-Z-Pamphlet"* **Diazepam** | *"Nitro-Z-Pamphlet"* **Nitrazepam** |

### Z-Drugs

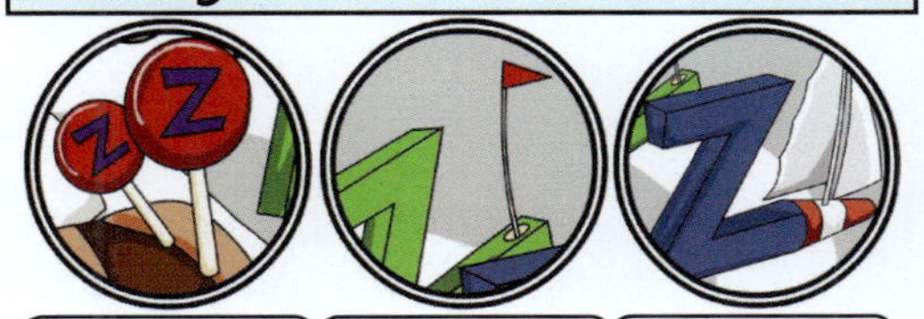

| | | |
|---|---|---|
| *"Z-POP"* **Zopiclone** | *"Z-Hole"* **Zolpidem** | *"Z-Sail-Pilon"* **Zaleplon** |

### Antidepressants

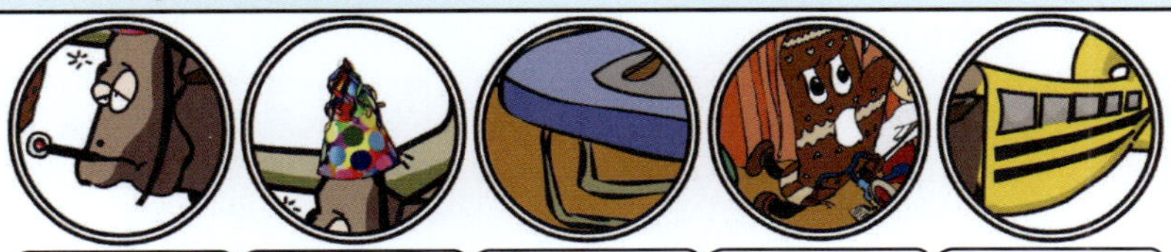

| | | | | |
|---|---|---|---|---|
| *"Flu-Ox"* **Fluoxetine** | *"Party-Ox"* **Paroxetine** | *"Trampoline"* **Sertraline** | *"A-Mitt-Trip"* **Amitriptyline** | *"Bus-Spirol"* **Buspirone** |

### Beta-Blockers

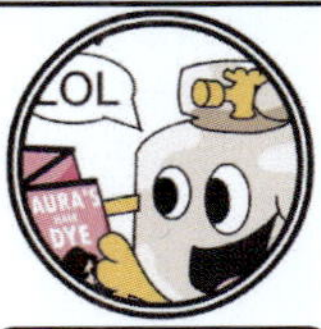

| |
|---|
| *"Propane-LOL"* **Propranolol** |

### Barbiturates

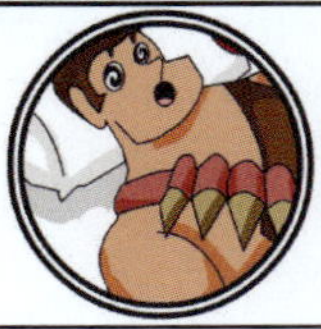

| |
|---|
| *"Ammo-Barbarian"* **Amobarbital** |

# ASTHMA

**Indications for asthma medications:** asthma, COPD.

**ASTHMA** is a chronic disease of the respiratory tract characterized by a triad of symptoms: hypersensitivity, airway inflammation, and reversible airway obstruction.

Asthma may be triggered by certain allergic or environmental factors and may also be associated with genetic factors. Treatment for asthma is aimed at reversing airway spasms and preventing hypersensitivity reactions by the use of relievers and controllers. Relievers are used to reverse an acute asthmatic attack, while controllers are used to prevent the occurrence of attacks.

Asthma is usually treated with a combination of B2-agonists and steroids, however, there are numerous second-line/adjunctive treatment options such as leukotriene receptor antagonists (LTRAs), phosphodiesterase (PDE) inhibitors, anticholinergic drugs, mast-cell stabilizers, and monoclonal antibodies.

## Beta 2-Receptor Agonists

All beta-2 agonists act by causing bronchodilation through smooth muscle relaxation in the lung.

***Salbutamol*** is a short acting beta 2-receptor agonists and is an example of a popular reliever. It has an onset of action of approximately fifteen minutes.

***Salmeterol*** and ***formoterol*** are long acting beta-2 agonists and are used as controllers. Their duration of effect lasts about twelve hours, providing a more stable airway patency throughout the day.

## Corticosteroids

In more severe cases where beta-2 agonists are not sufficient for asthma relief, corticosteroids may be added to the treatment regime.

***Budesonide*** and ***fluticasone*** are examples of corticosteroids used in asthma. Corticosteroids act by suppressing hypersensitivity type I reactions through the inhibition of the immune response. Adverse effects include thrush, cough, and hoarseness. For asthma sufferers, corticosteroids are usually administered by either inhalers or nebulizers, but where those have been unsuccessful, these can also be taken as an oral tablet.

## Leukotriene Receptor Antagonists (LRTAs)

***Montelukast*** is a LRTA that acts by blocking the action of leukotriene D4 on cysteinyl leukotriene receptors in the lungs and bronchial airways. Leukotrienes are inflammatory molecules that normally facilitate bronchospasms, so by blocking the action of these molecules, patients experience relief from chest tightness and shortness of breath.

## Phosphodiesterase (PDE) Inhibitors

***Theophylline*** is a PDE inhibitor that acts through competitive inhibition of phosphodiesterase, and leads to the inactivation of tumor necrosis factor (TNF)-alpha and the prevention of leukotriene synthesis. The clinical outcome is a relaxation of bronchial smooth muscles. Theophylline has a narrow therapeutic window, thus, small overdoses may lead to toxicity causing heart rate increase, abnormal heart rhythms, CNS excitation, and/or seizures.

## Anticholinergic Drugs

***Ipratropium*** is an anticholinergic drug that is used to relax and open up inflamed airways. The onset of their action is approximately fifteen minutes and effects last up to five hours. Ipratropium acts by blocking muscarinic receptors in bronchial airways to prevent acetylcholine from stimulating bronchoconstriction and mucus secretion.

## Mast-Cell Stabilizers

***Cromoglycate*** is a mast-cell stabilizer that prevents the release of histamine and other cytokines from mast cells. Cromoglycate is used for the prevention of allergic reactions or exercise-induced asthma, not for the treatment of acute asthmatic attacks.

## Monoclonal Antibodies (mAb)

***Omalizumab*** is a monoclonal antibody used for moderate to severe persistent asthma, whose symptoms are not controlled with inhaled corticosteroids. Omalizumab acts by binding to free IgE antibodies circulating in the bloodstream and thereby preventing hypersensitivity reactions from occurring. Omalizumab may cause anaphylaxis, a life-threatening systemic allergic reaction.

## Inhalers

This picture also highlights some of the most popular inhalers and their contents. Some inhalers, such as ***Ventolin*** (***salbutamol***) and ***Atrovent*** (***ipratropium***), administer only single agents. Whereas, inhalers can also contain a combination of drugs for administration, such as ***Seretide*** (***salmeterol*** and ***fluticasone***) and ***Symbicort*** (***formoterol*** and ***budesonide***).

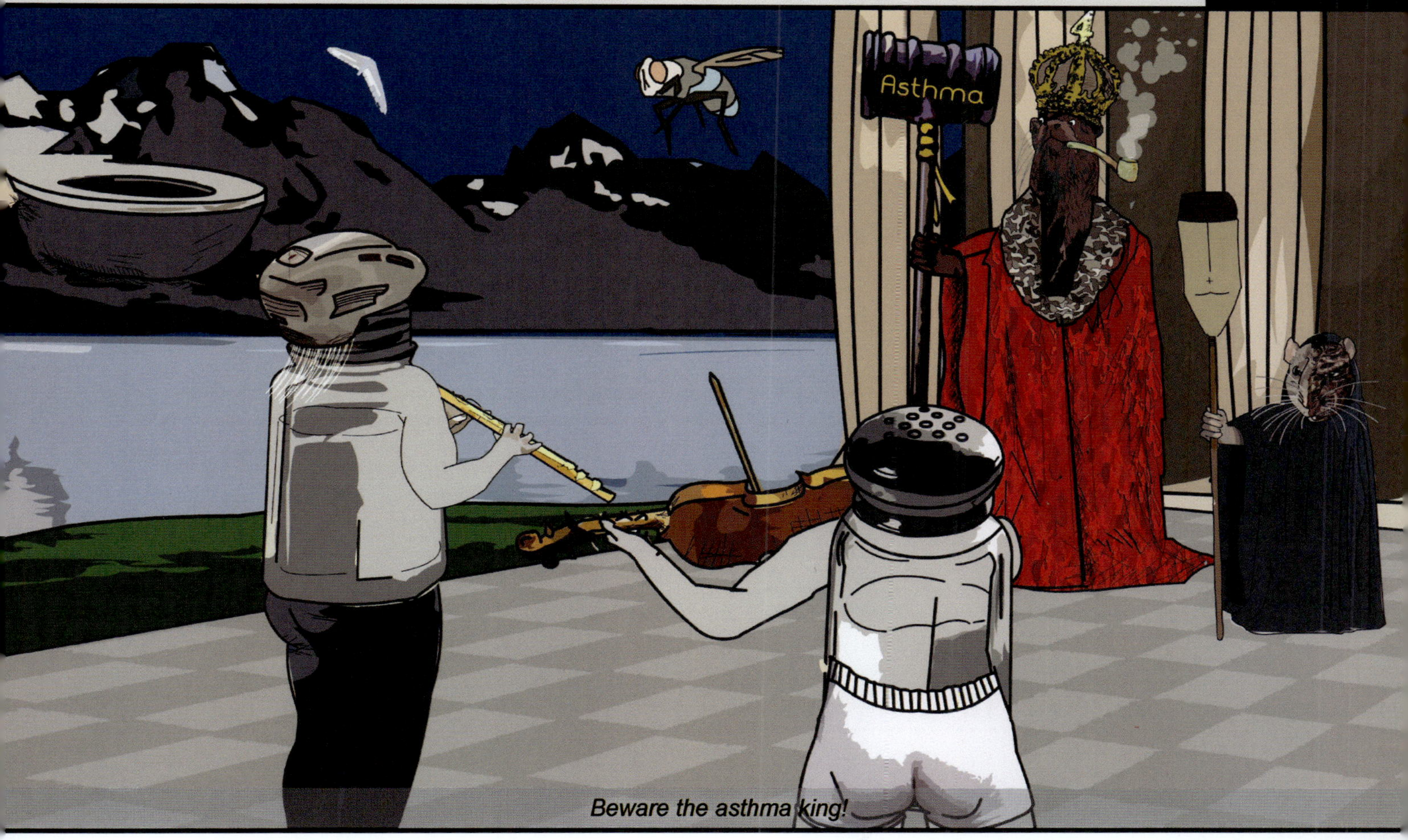


*Beware the asthma king!*

## ASTHMA

*The asthma king reminds you this picture is about asthma! Additionally, drugs are grouped with symbols that remind you of the name of their respective inhalers. Example: Salt-butt [salbutamol] playing the violin [Ventolin inhaler].*

### B2-Agonist

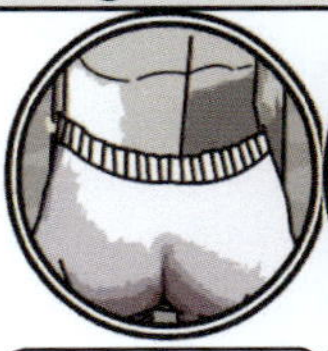

*"Salt-Butt"*
**Salbutamol**

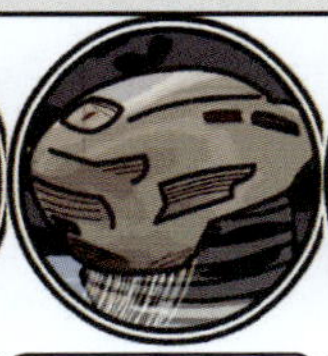

*"Salt-Helmet"*
**Salmeterol**

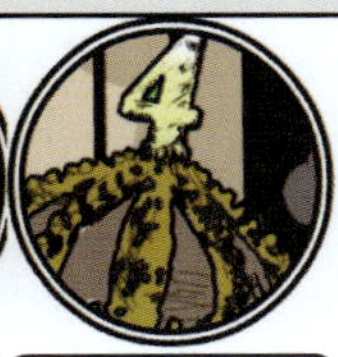


*"4"*
**Formoterol**

### Steroids

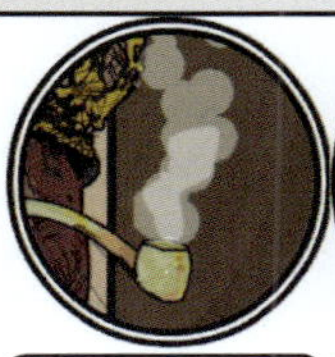

*"Bud"*
**Budesonide**

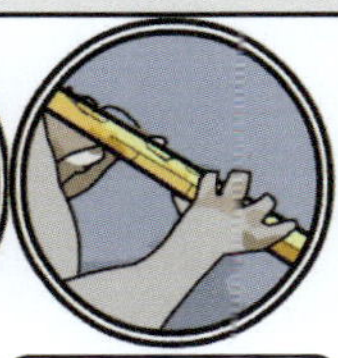

*"Flute"*
**Fluticascne**

### LTRA

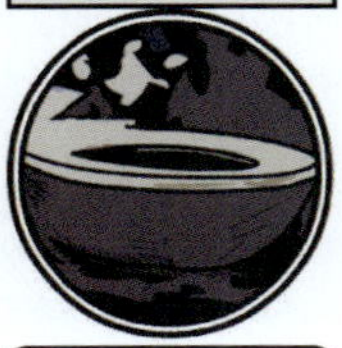

*"Mount-Loo"*
**Montelukast**

### PDE Inhibitors

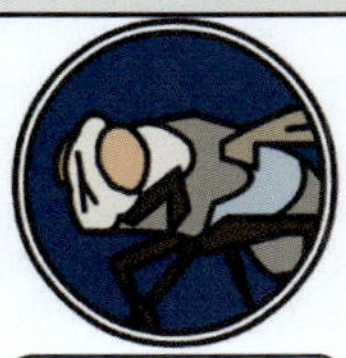

*"The-Fly"*
**Theophylline**

### Anticholinergic

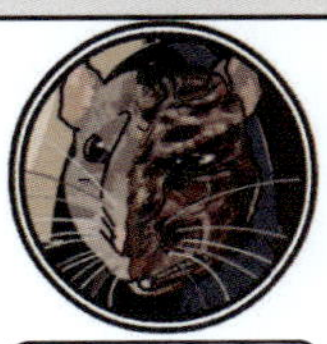

*"Rat"*
**Ipratropium**

### Mast-Cell Stabilizer

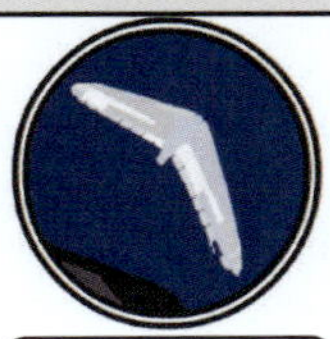

*"Chrome-Glyde"*
**Cromoglycate**

### mAb

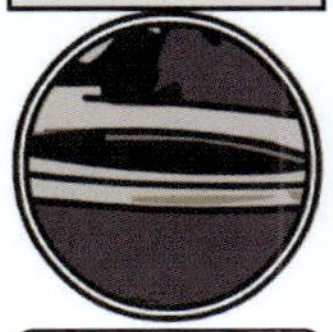

*"O-Lid"*
**Omalizumab**

### Inhalers

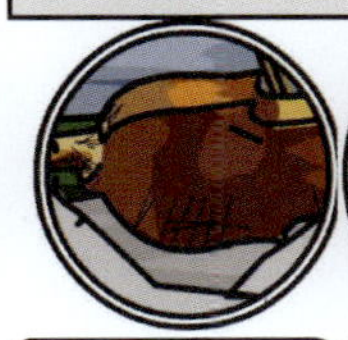

*"Violin"*
**Vento in**
*Contains Salbutamol*

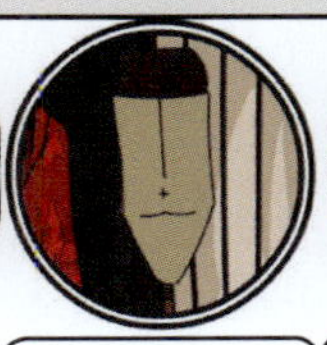

*"Row"*
**Atrovent**
*Contains Ipratropium*

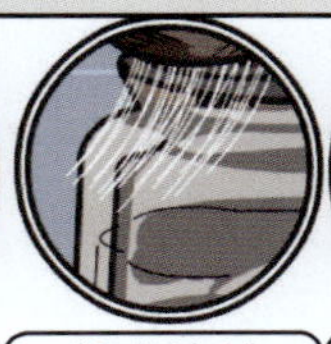

*"Salt-Hair"*
**Seretide**
*Contains Salmeterol and Fluticasone*

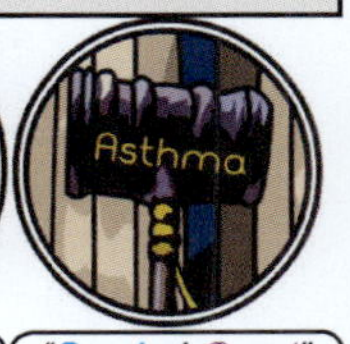


*"Symbol-Court"*
**Symbicort**
*Contains Formoterol and Budesonide*

# CANCER DRUGS

**Indications for cancer medications:** cancer.

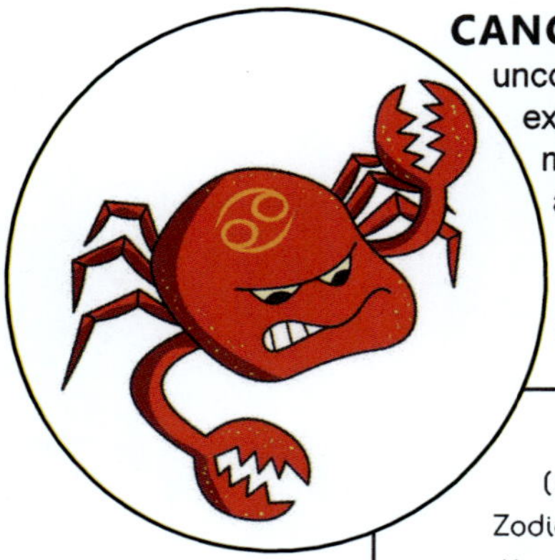

**CANCER** is characterized by mutational changes in cells within the body which may lead to uncontrollable proliferation. It can arise spontaneously, due to inherited factors, or due to exposure to extrinsic factors such as radiation and toxic chemical substances. Cancer cells may spread to other organs through the vascular or the lymphatic system. In turn, invasion and proliferation of cancerous cells into organs can eventually lead to organ failure.

Chemotherapy targets cancer cells by inhibiting important steps in cell division. Because cancer cells divide so quickly, they are more susceptible to these drugs.

The cancer symbol (astrological sign in the Zodiac) on the crab reminds you this picture is about cancer!

## Vinca Alkaloids

***Vinblastine*** and ***vincristine*** act by blocking the mitotic cycle of cancer cells and preventing cellular proliferation. They are used for the treatment of various types of cancer such as Hodgkin's lymphoma, non-small cell lung cancer, brain cancer, skin cancer, and testicular cancer. Some side effects of this drug class include headache, weakness, and anorexia. In rare cases, it can lead to cytopenia and shortness of breath.

## Antimetabolites

***Methotrexate***, ***fluorouracil***, and ***mercaptopurine***, are antimetabolites that inhibit DNA synthesis in cancer cells.

***Methotrexate*** is used in the treatment of breast, head, neck, lung, and bladder cancer. It can also be used to treat leukemia, lymphoma, and osteosarcoma. Methotrexate acts as a competitive inhibitor of dihydrofolate reductase, an enzyme required for the synthesis of tetrahydrofolate. The end result is the inhibition of folic acid synthesis and a failure of DNA and RNA synthesis within the cancer cell. Similar to vinca alkaloids, methotrexate has been associated with severe cytopenia and increased risk of infection.

***Fluorouracil*** acts as an inhibitor of thymidylate synthase, which is an enzyme required in the synthesis of pyrimidine thymidine, a nucleoside required for DNA replication. Therefore, by blocking this process, DNA replication is halted in the cancer cell. Fluorouracil is usually administered intravenously to treat colon, esophageal, pancreatic, and cervical cancer. Fluorouracil also comes in the form of topical cream which can be used to treat basal cell carcinoma, a form of skin cancer associated with long periods of exposure to sun.

***Mercaptopurine*** prevents the formation of DNA and RNA in cancer cells by disrupting the cascade involved in purine synthesis. It is used to treat various cancers, including leukemia, but can also be used for autoimmune conditions such as Crohn's disease and ulcerative colitis.

## Alkylating Agents

***Cyclophosphamide***, ***carboplatin***, ***cisplatin***, and ***busulfan***'s chemotherapeutic and cytotoxic effects come from their ability for alkylation and cross linking of DNA. This interferes with the ability of DNA strands to separate during replication. Cyclophosphamide is the most widely used alkylating agent and is used for the treatment of cancers such as leukemia, lymphoma, multiple myeloma, and ovarian cancer among others. Furthermore, it has also been used to treat autoimmune diseases where DMARDs have failed. Common side effects include nausea and vomiting, bone marrow suppression, and increased risk of bleeding from the bladder.

## Taxanes

***Paclitaxel*** works by causing defects in mitotic spindle assembly, chromosome segregation, and cell division. It is used for the treatment of various types of cancers including skin, prostate, lung, and bladder cancer. It is also effective against Kaposi sarcoma, a medical complication in AIDS patients. The use of paclitaxel may lead to side effects such as bone marrow suppression, numbness of the limbs, muscle aches, and hair loss.

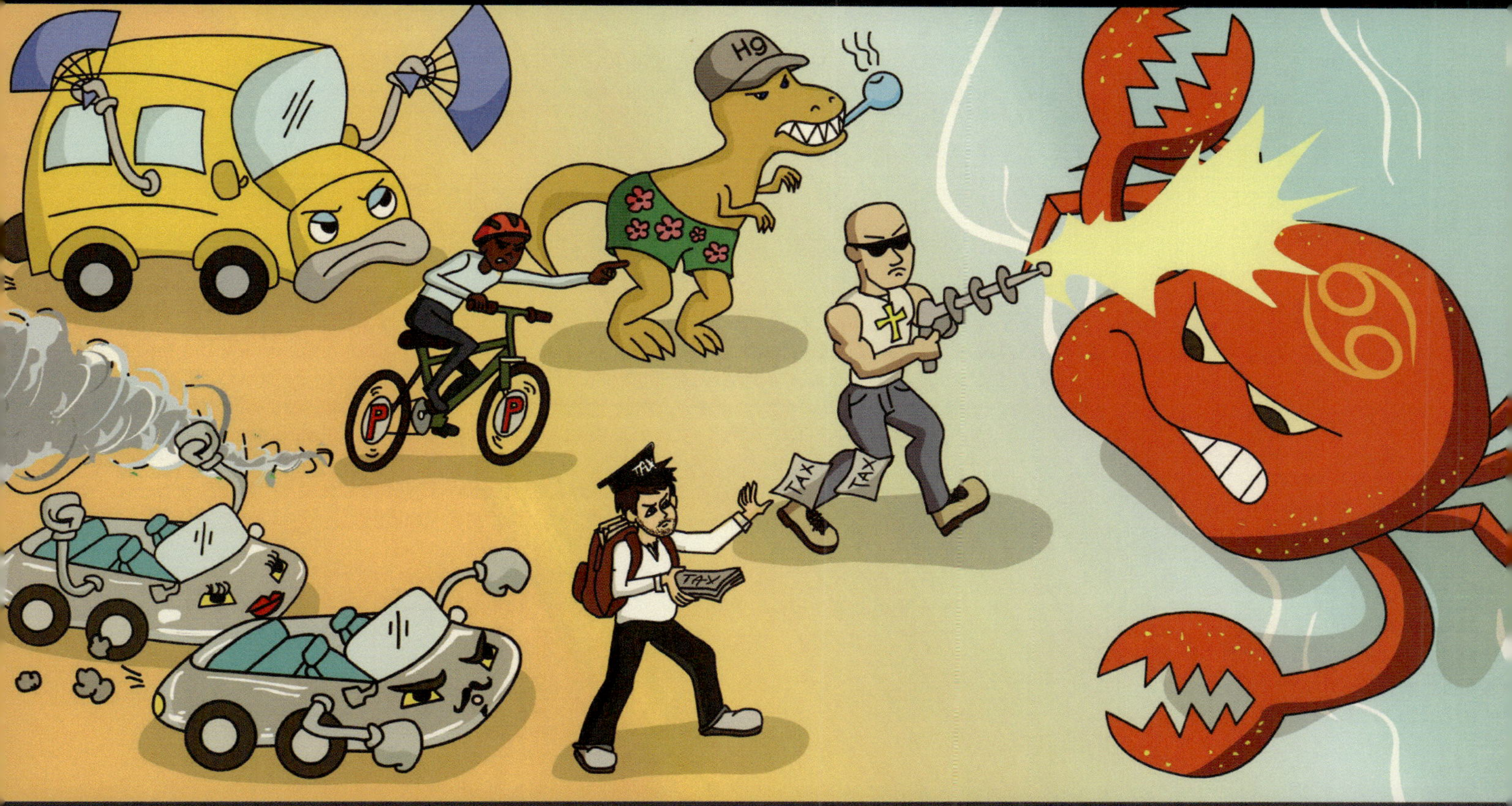


Kill the cancer crab!

## CANCER DRUGS

*The cancer symbol (astrological sign in the Zodiac) on the crab reminds you this picture is about cancer!*

### Vinca Alkaloids

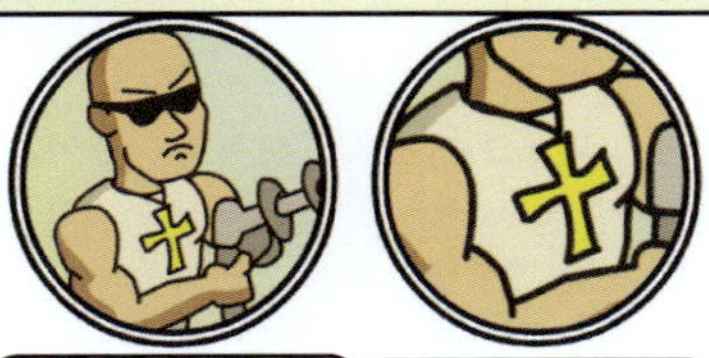

- *"Vin-Blasting"* **Vinblastine**
- *"Vin-Cross"* **Vincristine**

### Antimetabolites

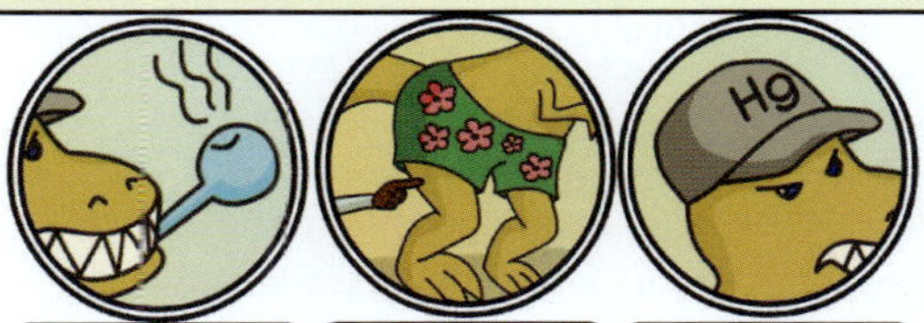


- *"Meth-T-Rex"* **Methotrexate**
- *"Floral"* **Fluorouracil**
- *"Mercury-Cap"* **Mercaptopurine** *[Mercury is Hg on periodic table]*

### Alkylating Agents

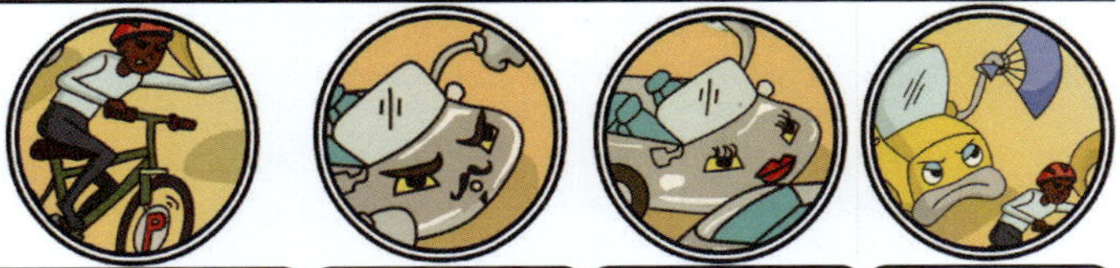

- *"Cycle-Phosphate"* **Cyclophosphamide**
- *"Car-Platinum"* **Carboplatin**
- *"Sis-Platinum"* **Cisplatin**
- *"Bus-Fan"* **Busulfan**

### Taxanes

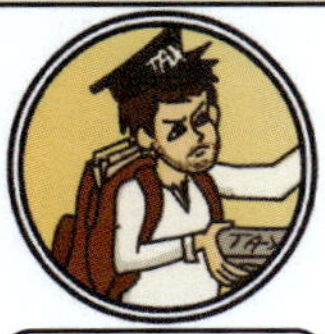

- *"Pack-Tax"* **Paclitaxel**

# RHEUMATOID ARTHRITIS

**Indications for antirheumatic drugs:** autoimmune diseases (RA, SLE, etc.).

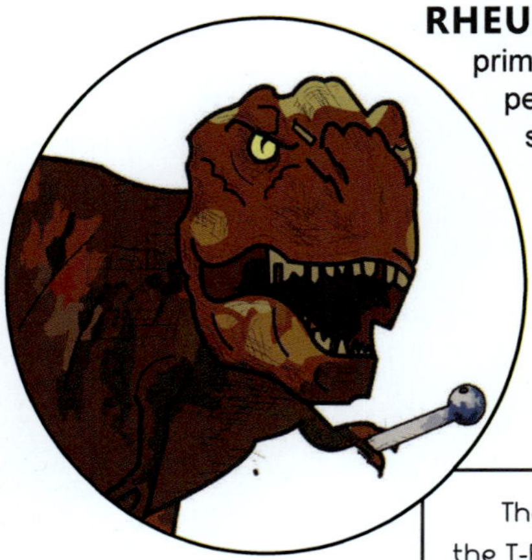


**RHEUMATOID ARTHRITIS (RA)** is a chronic inflammatory autoimmune disease that primarily affects the joints. People who suffer from RA usually complain of symmetrical and persistent joint pain in the upper and lower limbs, some of which will present with bone structure deformities. The wrist, proximal interphalangeal (PIP) and metacarpophalangeal (MCP) joints in the upper limb, and the metatarsophalangeal (MTP) joints in the lower limbs, are the most commonly affected joints. The goal of treatment is to slow down the progression of disease, relieve pain, and prevent complications.

Disease modifying anti-rheumatic drugs (DMARDs) are the main treatment for RA, and they are combined together with additional therapies such as corticosteroids and analgesics.

## Disease Modifying Anti-Rheumatic Drugs (DMARDs)

DMARDs are categorized into non-biological and biological by their molecular nature. The biological DMARDs are further sub-classified into the tumor necrosis factor (TNF) inhibitors and non-TNF inhibitors. Ultimately, these drugs work by suppressing the immune system and decreasing the inflammatory response in targeted joints.

## Non-Biological

***Methotrexate*** is a non-biologic DMARD used in the treatment of various cancers, and in autoimmune diseases like rheumatoid arthritis, psoriasis, and Crohn's disease. As an antimetabolite, it inhibits the enzymes responsible for the synthesis of T-lymphocytes (immune cells responsible for cell-mediated immune response) and prevents the binding of interleukin 1-beta to its surface receptor which suppresses inflammatory processes. Methotrexate can also disrupt bone marrow production of cells, which may lead to an increased chance of infection and bleeding and furthermore, can cause liver damage. It is recommended that individuals abstain from alcohol while taking this medication.

***Leflunomide***, another non-biologic DMARD, is an immunosuppressive drug that acts by inhibiting an enzyme called dihydroorotate dehydrogenase and prevents the synthesis of DNA and RNA in rapidly dividing cells. It is used primarily for rheumatoid arthritis and side effects include temporary hair loss, rash, and liver damage.

***Gold salts*** have an unknown mechanism of action for rheumatoid arthritis. Its use has decreased substantially over the last twenty years due to numerous side effects and the need for monitoring.

***Hydroxychloroquine*** was originally used to treat malaria, but later was seen to help with symptoms of arthritis and is often used in combination with other DMARDS.

***Sulfasalazine*** is used to treat rheumatoid arthritis, along with arthritis associated with inflammatory bowel disease. Sulfasalazine may cause an interesting side effect in that it can cause urine, sweat, and tears to have an orange color.

## Biological TNF-Inhibitors

TNF-inhibitors include medications like soluble receptor antagonists, such as ***etanercept***, and monoclonal antibodies, such as ***adalimumab*** and ***infliximab***. These medications bind to cytokines, including TNF, a molecule involved in the inflammatory response and joint problems associated with rheumatoid arthritis, and prevent them from interacting with cell receptors.

## Non TNF-Inhibitors

***Abatacept*** is an immune suppressing non-TNF inhibiting drug. It acts by blocking antigen presenting cells (APC) from delivering co-stimulatory signals needed for cell mediated immune responses. In turn, this prevents T-lymphocytes from fully activating and downregulates the inflammatory response.

***Rituximab*** is a non-TNF inhibiting biologic that binds to an antigen called CD-20 located on the surface of immature B-lymphocytes. This leads to antibody-dependent cellular cytotoxicity (ADCC), complement-dependent cytotoxicity (CDC), and an induction of cell degeneration by means of apoptosis.

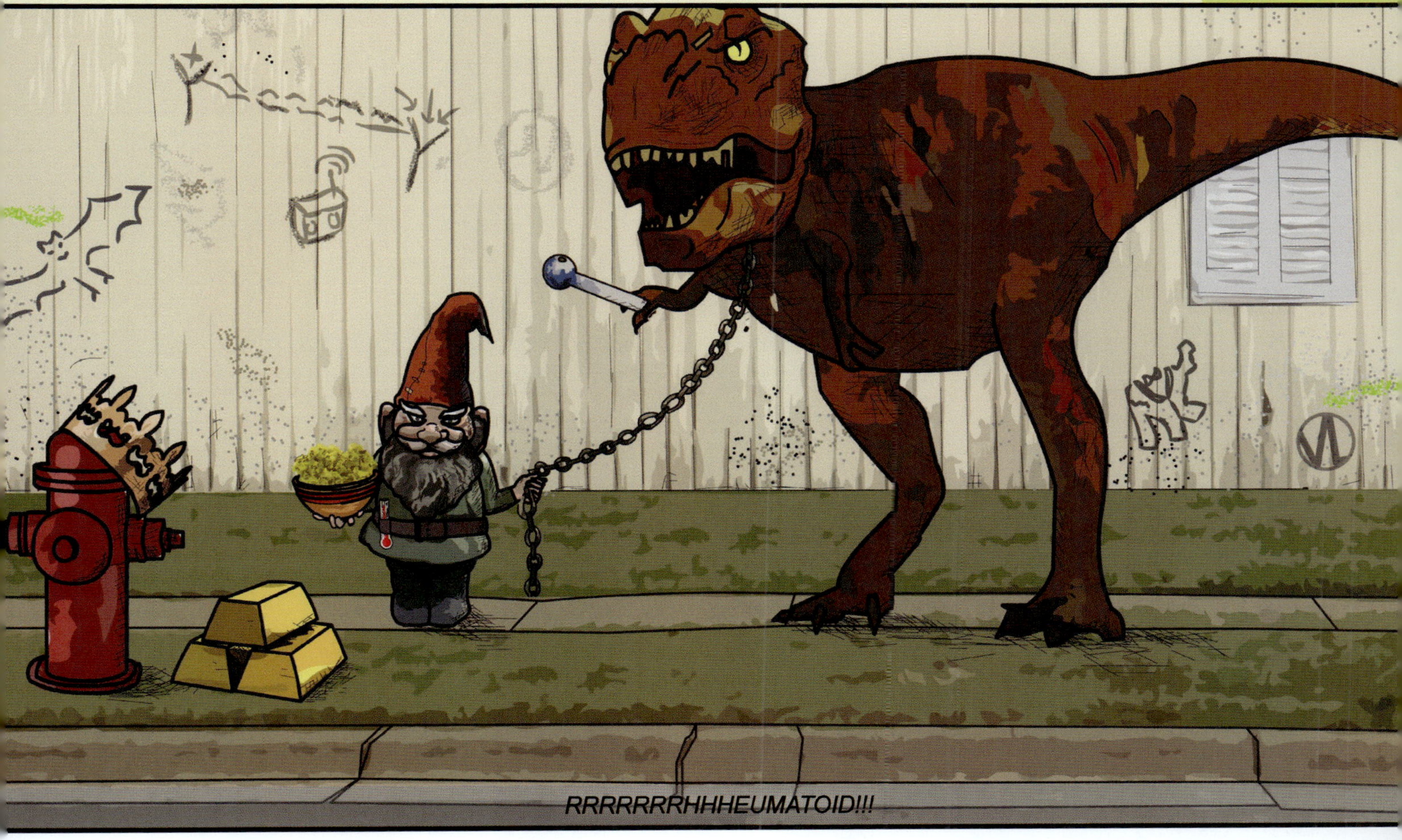


## RHEUMATOID ARTHRITIS

*The "RRRRRROAAAAR" of the T-Rex will remind you of RRRRRRRHEUMATOID!*

### DMARDS

### Non-Biological

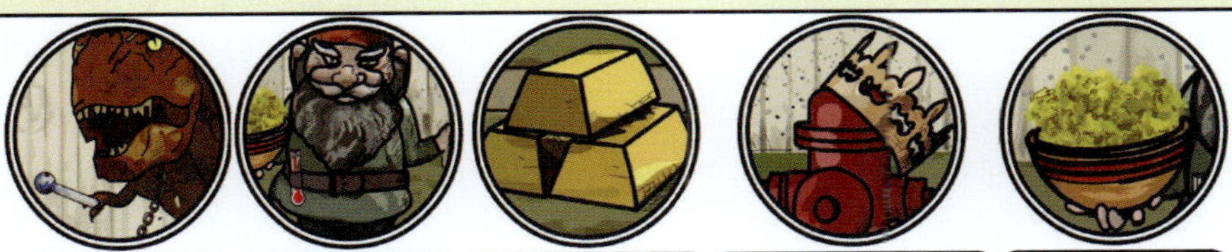

| "Meth-T-Rex" | "Flu-Gnome" | "Gold" | "Hydro-Queen" | "Sulfur-Salad" |
|---|---|---|---|---|
| **Methotrexate** | **Leflunomide** | **Gold Salts** | **Hydroxychloroquine** | **Sulfasalazine** |

### Biological

#### TNF Inhibitors

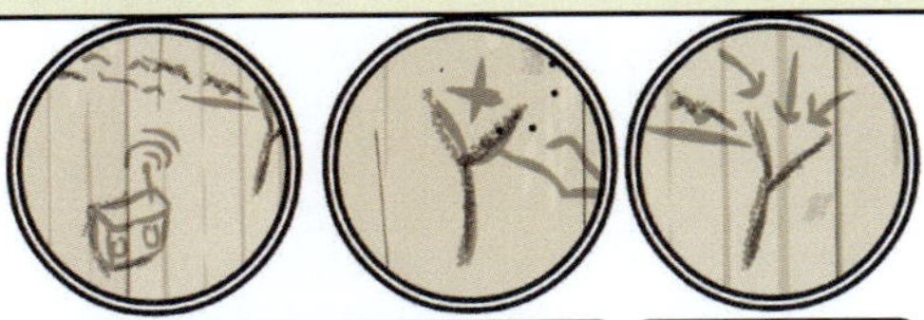

| "Intercept" | "Add-mAb" | "Influx-mAb" |
|---|---|---|
| **Etanercept** | **Adalimumab** | **Infliximab** |

#### Non-TNF Inhibitors

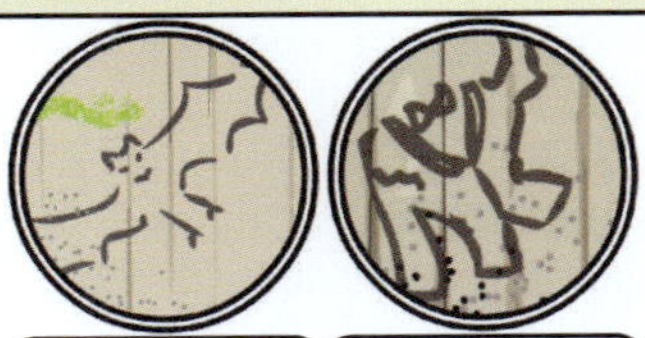

| "A-Bat" | "Ripped-Tux" |
|---|---|
| **Abatacept** | **Rituximab** |

*mAb is short for monoclonal antibody, which is often depicted in the shape of a Y.*

# DRUG MISUSE AND DEPENDANCE

**Indications:** various drugs of abuse are used as medical treatments, for example, benzodiazepines are used for anxiety disorders.

**THERE ARE A RANGE OF MEDICATIONS** and substances that are being misused due to their ability to cause euphoria, unfortunately, some of these drugs can also cause physical and psychological dependence. Substances of abuse are categorised into general depressants, opioids, stimulants, hallucinogens, and some that are unique and do not fit into conventional categories.

## General Depressants

Central nervous system (CNS) depressants are drugs that slow down neurotransmission in the brain and consist of benzodiazepines, barbiturates, and alcohol.

***Benzodiazepines*** treat anxiety, acute stress reactions, and panic attacks. They act by enhancing the inhibitory effect of gamma-aminobutyric acid (GABA) by binding to the $GABA_A$ receptor, a chloride channel found on neurons, and increasing the rate of opening. This hyperpolarizes the neuron by allowing more chloride to enter the cell, making firing less likely. These actions account for the anxiolytic, sedative, and muscle relaxing effects of benzodiazepines.

Similarly to benzodiazepines, ***barbiturates*** bind to $GABA_A$ receptors and potentiate their inhibitory effects. Instead of increasing the rate of opening of the $GABA_A$ receptor chloride channel, they increase the duration of opening to hyperpolarize the neuron.

***Alcohol*** is another CNS depressant which binds to $GABA_A$ receptors allowing chloride to flow more freely through its channel and potentiating the inhibitory effects of GABA. As with benzodiazepines and barbiturates, long term consumption of alcohol will lead to dependence and withdrawal symptoms such as nausea, vomiting, headache, sweating, palpitations, and anorexia.

## Opioids

Opioids are psychoactive substances derived from poppy plants that are medically used for analgesia, but also produce a strong euphoria. Some examples of opioids include ***diamorphine*** (also known as heroin, see alternative character in opioid chapter on page 13), ***morphine***, and ***pethidine***.

Opioids bind to the opioid receptors, which are primarily located in the central and peripheral nervous systems. Methadone and buprenorphine are longer acting opioids that may be used as substitutes for diamorphine addiction and can help in the detoxification process.

## Stimulants

Stimulant drugs produce an increase in wakefulness, energy, sexual arousal, and a greater sense of euphoria. Examples include ***amphetamine***, ***3,4-methylenedioxymethamphetamine (MDMA)***, and ***cocaine***. Side effects include acute psychosis, hepatotoxicity, cardiotoxicity, jaw clenching, and tooth grinding.

***Cocaine*** acts by preventing the reuptake of neurotransmitters such as epinephrine, norepinephrine, and serotonin which results in an increase in neuronal activity in the synaptic cleft. It has a rapid onset of action (seconds), especially after inhalation.

***Amphetamines*** lead to intracellular release of various catecholamines (serotonin, norepinephrine, and dopamine) into the synaptic cleft, and also decrease the metabolism of these catecholamines. This causes these neurotransmitters to exert their effects on postsynaptic neurons for longer periods of time and to a greater extent. Traditionally, amphetamines are used to treat attention deficit hyperactivity disorder (ADHD) and narcolepsy. MDMA, often referred to as ecstasy, is another stimulant which exhibits its effect in the same way as amphetamines and is also used to treat ADHD.

## Hallucinogens

Hallucinogens are a group of psychoactive substances that can induce hallucinations, false imaginary perceptions and changes in behavior, emotions, and consciousness. They bind and activate postsynaptic serotonin receptors which leads to an increase in brain activity and altered awareness to the surroundings. Examples of hallucinogens include ***lysergic acid diethylamide*** (***LSD***), ***psilocybin mushroom***, and ***dimethyltryptamine*** (***DMT***).

## Other Commonly Abused Substances

***Nicotine*** is a drug found in cigarettes and cigars, and has both stimulant and depressant properties. It acts as an agonist at nicotinic receptors, leading to the release of many chemical messengers in the brain and cause feelings of relaxation, sharpness, and calmness.

***Marijuana***, otherwise known as cannabis, is derived from a flowering plant in the Cannabaceae family. The pharmacologically active metabolite is tetrahydrocannabinol (THC), which exerts its effects by binding to the cannabinoid receptors on neurons in the brain. Acute effects include euphoria and anxiety.

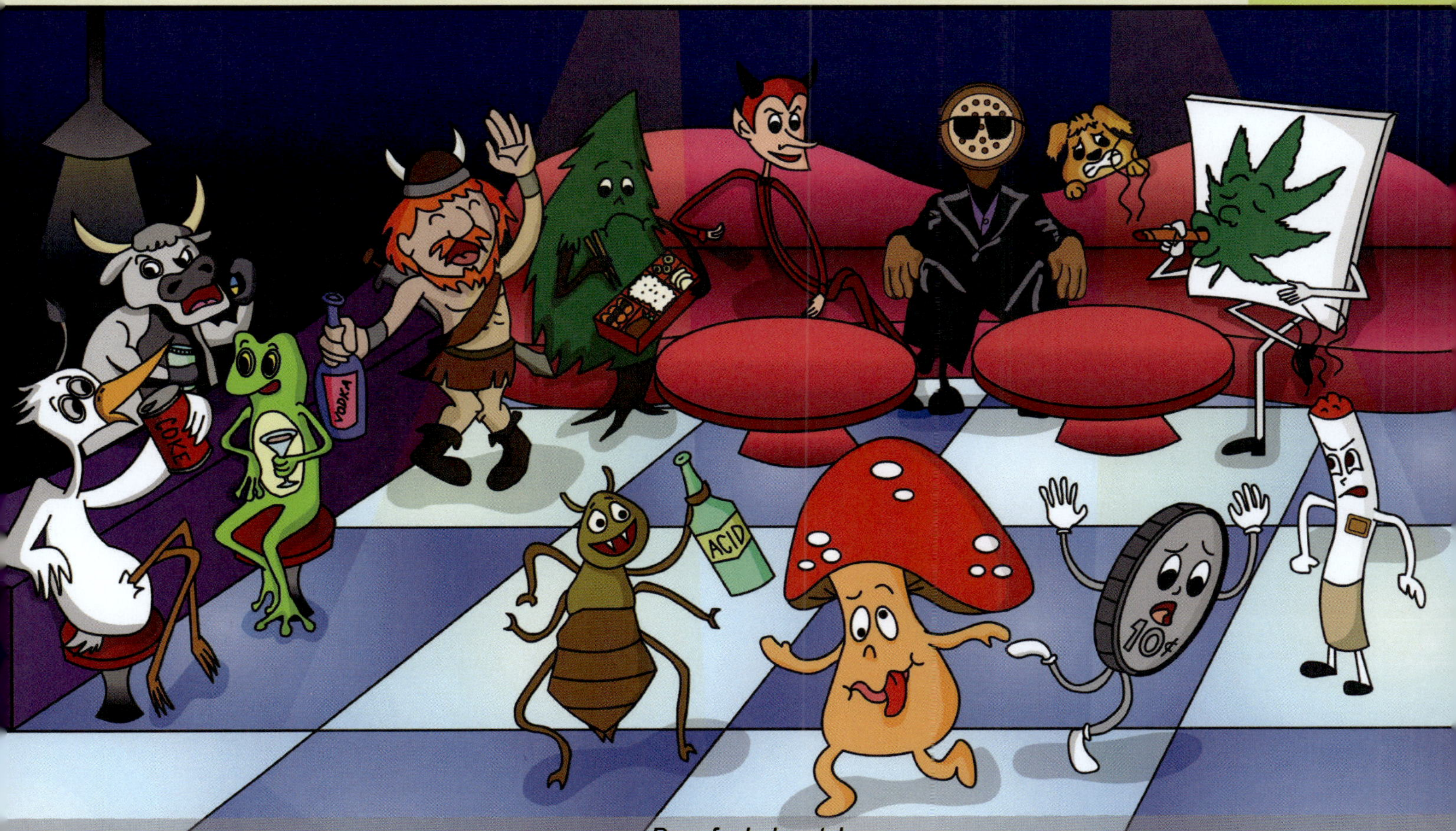


*Drug fueled party!*

## DRUG MISUSE AND DEPENDENCE

*All the Illicit drugs used at this party will remind you that this picture is about drug misuse and dependence!*

### General Depressants

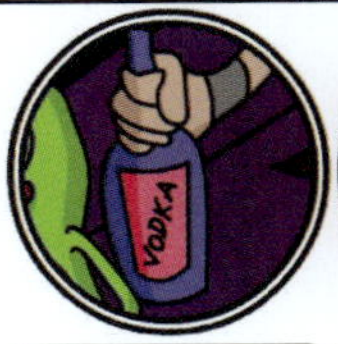


*"Alcohol"*
**Alcohol**

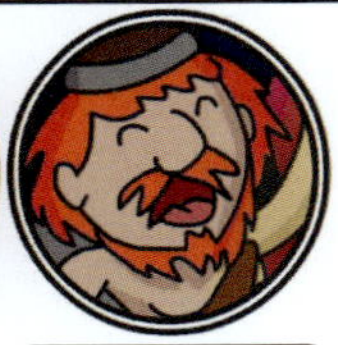

*"Barbarian"*
**Barbituates**

### Benzodiazepines

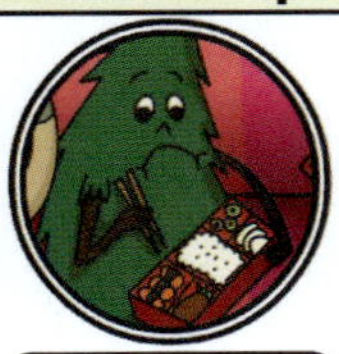

*"Bento-Pine"*
**Benzodiazepines**

### Opioids

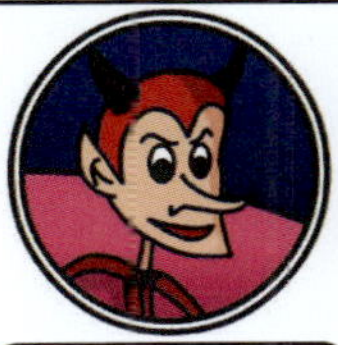

*"Devil-Fiend"*
**Diamorphine**
(Heroin)

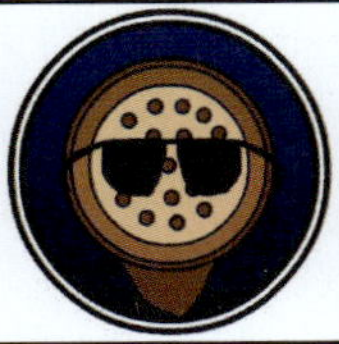

*"Morpheus-Phone"*
**Morphine**

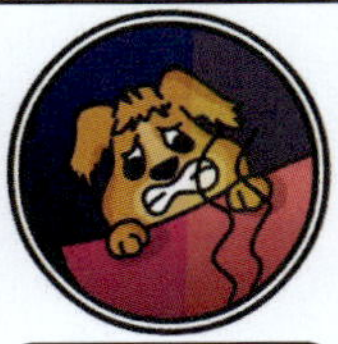

*"Pet-Hiding"*
**Pethidine**

### Stimulants

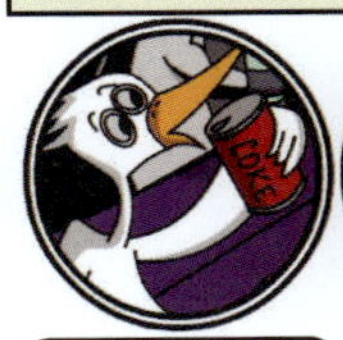


*"Coke-Crane"*
**Cocaine**

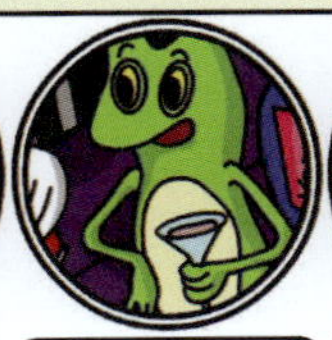

*"Amphibian"*
**Amfetamines**

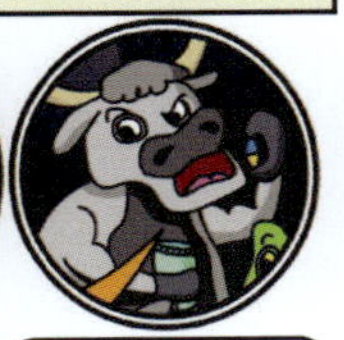

*"Metal-Ox"*
**Methylenedioxy-**
Methamphetamine
(Ecstacy)

### Hallucinogens

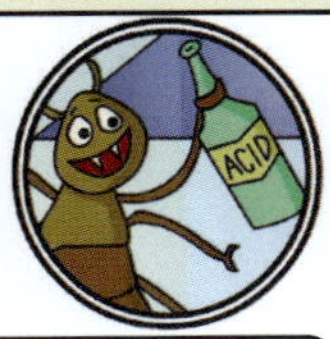


*"Lice-Acid"*
**Lysergic Acid**
Diethylamide
(LSD)

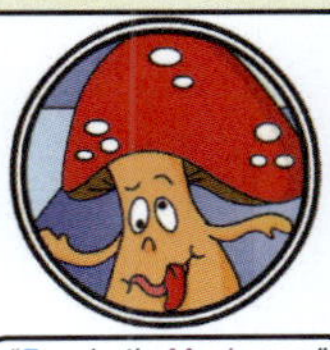

*"Psychotic Mushroom"*
**Psilocybin Mushroom**
(Psilocin)

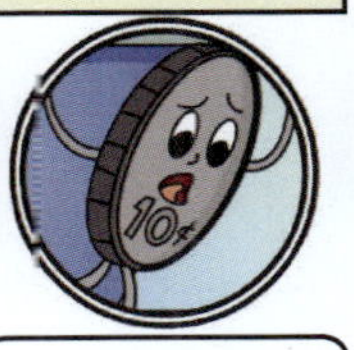


*"Dime-Trip"*
**Dimethyl-tryptamine**

### Other

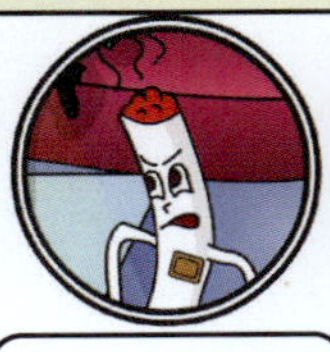

*"Nicotine [Patch]"*
**Nicotine**

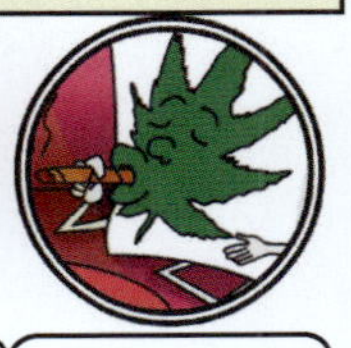

*"Marijuana"*
**Marijuana**

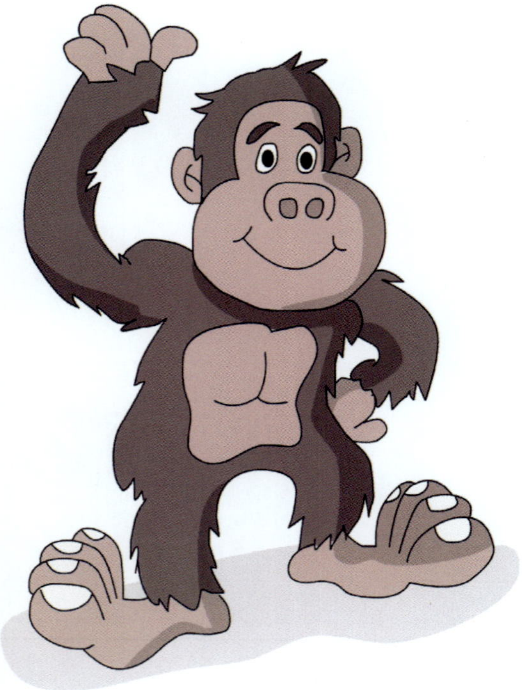

25452769R00056

Printed in Poland
by Amazon Fulfillment
Poland Sp. z o.o., Wrocław